What Your Doctor Never Told You About...

{ Aches, Strains, and Back Pains }

What Your Doctor Never Told You About...

{ Aches, Strains, and Back Pains }

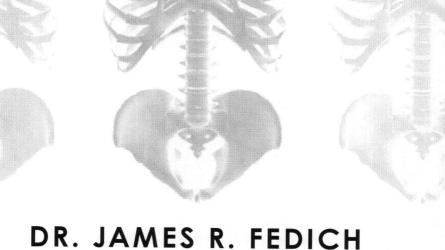

DR. JAMES R. FEDICH

Intro:

Starfish Story

A Buddhist monk was walking along the shore with a disciple the morning after a terrible storm. There were several starfishes trapped on the beach; they would certainly die if left out in the harsh sun.

The monk bent down, picked one up and threw it back into the ocean. His disciple looked puzzled and asked him why he would do this when there were miles of beached starfish lying out in the sun. It can't possibly make a significant difference, he reasoned. The monk quietly picked up the next one and said to the disciple "It makes a difference to this one" and threw it into the ocean as well.

Do what you can for the people around you; it may not change the whole world, but it will change that one person's world.

This book was written on just that principle. It is my hope that through reading this book, you can come to a greater understanding of the human form as it relates to the back and nerves, and that you will be able to see the importance of chiropractic work in the lives of the people. If a chiropractor can help just one person to be able to walk freely and comfortably again, then their job is done.

About Dr. Fedich

YEARS AGO SOMETHING happened to me that **changed my life forever.** *Let me tell you my story.*

Back in the eighth grade I was taking a family trip to a wedding in beautiful upstate New York. We were driving along, my mother, father, my brother, and I, on some back roads. The weather was lovely; everyone was enjoying the drive, and then.... CRASH!

Out of nowhere, a young woman ran a stop sign and hit our car at 45 mph. Next thing I knew, I was in a hospital on a backboard. I returned home, only to realize that I had agonizing back pain all day long. I could barely get off the floor. I couldn't play basketball anymore, and that is all I lived for. I remember lying on the floor, *in crippling pain,* not being able to get up using my own power. I was forced to lie on my back for eight hours and wait for my parents to get home from work to help me up. The pain was debilitating; I thought that I would never play basketball again. What agonizing pain. *But, there's more...*

My mother decided to take me to a new doctor. This new doctor did an exam, took some films, and then 'adjusted' my spine. The adjustment didn't hurt, it actually felt good, I got relief. *Oh, did I mention that this doctor is a chiropractor?* Within two weeks I was back playing basketball for my team again. It worked so well for me, and I was so impressed with the other 'miracles' I saw in his office, that *I* eventually went to chiropractic school myself. I have been helping patients with their problems for ten years now, and I love being able to give back the gift that I received from my chiropractor many years ago. I grew up in Long Valley, New Jersey, only fifteen minutes away from my office. It's great to return to the area I grew up and be able to give back to the community.

After graduating high school, I went on to receive by Bachelor of Science degree, with honors, from the University of Hartford, in Connecticut, and I did it in only three years. After receiving my Bachelor's degree, I continued on to receive my Doctor of Chiropractic degree from New York Chiropractic College in Seneca Falls, NY. I also graduated with high honors and was inducted into the Phi Chi Omega scholastic honor society.

After receiving my Doctorate from NYCC, I began work in one of the largest sports medicine clinics in the state of New Jersey. In Newark, I worked with an amazing interdisciplinary team including acupuncture, chiropractic, medical care, and neurology. I learned many things during my stay there, and I eventually branched out on my own in Allamuchy, New Jersey, which is 40 miles northwest of New York City, in the scenic Warren County of New Jersey. I have been committed to helping people the way I was helped, in addition to writing and consulting as well. I am currently a state Board of Directors member for the Association of New Jersey Chiropractors. It is the largest state chiropractic association in the country, and one of the largest chiropractic associations in the world, with over 2,000 members. I sit on the board of twelve who make decisions for our profession in the state of New Jersey and have national influence. I continue to run a full time practice in Allamuchy, New Jersey as well as working with interdisciplinary providers including pain management, physiatrist, and orthopedic surgeons in Hackettstown, New Jersey, and West Orange, New Jersey. In addition, I have written several health articles and do ergonomic and safety consulting for companies such as UPS in Mount Olive, New Jersey. I am also a consultant and author for the Nutritional Magnesium Association, http: *www.nutritionalmagnesium.org*.

More information about me or my activities can be found on our website at http://www.villagefamilychiro.com

CHAPTER 1

History of Spinal Problems

MAN'S STYLE OF WALKING is different than most, if not all, other mammals in the world. This refers to the fact that man walks on two feet rather than the biologically expected four feet, like other vertebrates. In this position, man is placed under stress unusual to most mammals, not only in that gravity pulls on the spine, but also in that anything carried by man is usually carried on the back or in the arms. This places an added strain on our spine, spreading to the rest of our joints.

Studies indicate that 80% of people in the United States will suffer some form of debilitating back pain in their lifetimes. This is in sharp contrast to some other cultures around the world, where back pain is present in less than 5% of the population. Noelle Perez, of the Institute D'Aplomb in Paris, conducted extensive research into the differences in lifestyle, which might be related to back pain.

The common thread in Portugal, Costa Rica, Bali and other countries with low incidence of back and joint pain is simple.

People have different posture than we, in the U.S, do. And as a result they have little or no back and joint pain. These people stand, sit and move slightly differently than we do, in a way that does not produce the tension that so many of us feel in our backs. The solution to your back pain is an adjustment in posture to a more natural way of standing.

The human body has evolved to support its weight through the skeleton. While this seems obvious, if you are reading this from the United States, the chances are your muscles are chronically doing extra work to support your body. Contrast these postures: a person with no back pain has their spine, pelvic center, knees and ankle naturally aligned as if on a plumb line, efficiently supporting their weight on solid bone. A person with typical posture in the United States is another story. It is definitely not uncommon to see Americans "slumping" around, with their shoulders bent, forcing their eyes to the ground. No, I'm not speaking primarily of older Americans, but rather the majority of Americans. If Americans would take better care to not only correct their own posture, but to instill the importance of proper posture into the minds of the young in the country, many back, knee, and other joint problems could be avoided.

To clearly see the difference, look at people in countries such as Portugal and Bali, who do not suffer from back pain. Their natural standing posture is erect and in line, and as a result, they suffer from very little back and joint pain. They have pain from diseases, poor diets, and accidents, but everyday movements like gardening, sitting, carrying children, sneezing or bending do not produce pain.

How did our society become so debilitated? The answer is a matter of historical record, as evidenced by photographs and medical records. Before the 1920's people in the United States stood with their spine, pelvis and legs on the same axis, with their body weight upright and vertical. In the 1920's, there was a shift in fashion. Think of the posture of the flappers. They stood stylishly, with their pelvis shifted forward. This modern look slowly influenced posture throughout our society, to the point where most people consider normal posture as being a lopsided awkward stance. Unfortunately, it has brought with it the raft of problems described above. Proper posture can help you unlearn the fashionable posture, and allow your body to heal its pain.

Back pain (also known as "dorsalgia") is pain felt in the back that usually originates from the muscles, nerves, bones, joints or other structures in the spine.

The pain can often be divided into neck pain, upper back pain, lower back pain or tailbone pain. It may have a sudden onset or can be a chronic pain; it can be constant or intermittent, stay in one place or radiate to other areas. It may be a dull ache, or a sharp or piercing or burning sensation. The pain may be radiated into the arm and hand, in the upper back, or in the low back, (and might radiate into the leg or foot), and may include symptoms other than pain, such as weakness, numbness or tingling.

Back pain is one of humanity's most frequent complaints. In the U.S., acute low back pain (also called lumbago) is the fifth most common reason for physician visits. About nine out of ten adults experience back pain at some point in their life, and five out of ten working adults have back pain every year.

Back pain is a common problem that affects most people at some stage in their lifetime. The back is prone to a range of problems including postural stress, muscle strains, ligament sprains, disc problems, sciatica, arthritis, structural defects, disease and fracture.

CHAPTER 2

Anatomy 101
the Spine, Vertebra, Discs

THE BACK IS AN INTRICATE STRUCTURE of interlocking components. Vertebrae are the bones that stack on top of each other
to make up the spinal column and protect the spinal cord.

A Vertebra

A typical vertebra has a drum-shaped "body" (centrum) that
forms a thick, anterior portion of the bone. A longitudinal row
of the bodies supports the weight of the head and trunk. The
intervertebral disks, which separate joining vertebrae, are fas-
tened to the roughened upper and lower surfaces of the bodies.
These disks cushion and soften the forces created by walking
and jumping, which might otherwise fracture the vertebrae or
jar the brain. Each intervertebral disk is composed of a band of
fibrous fibrocartilage (anulus fibrosus) that surrounds a gelati-
nous core, called the "nucleus pulposus." The bodies of adjacent
vertebrae are joined on the front surfaces by "anterior ligaments"
and on the back by "posterior ligaments."

Projecting from the back of each body are two short stalks called "pedicles." They form the sides of the "vertebral foramen." Two plates (laminae) arise from the pedicles and fuse in the back to become "spinous process." The pedicles, laminae, and spinous process together complete a bony vertebral arch around the vertebral opening, through which the spinal cord passes. Between the pedicles and laminae of a typical vertebra is a "transverse process" that projects laterally and toward the back.

Various ligaments and muscles are attached to the spinal process and the transverse process. Projecting upward and downward from each vertebral arch are "superior" and "inferior articulating processes." These processes bear cartilage-covered facets by which each vertebra is joined to the one above and the one below it. On the surfaces of the vertebral pedicles are notches that align to create openings, called "intervertebral foramina." These openings provide passageways for spinal nerves that proceed between joining vertebrae and connect to the spinal cord.

The spine is a column of vertebrae that supports the entire upper body. The column is grouped into three sections: the cervical vertebrae are the seven spinal bones that support the neck; the thoracic vertebrae are the twelve spinal bones that connect to the rib cage; and the lumbar vertebrae are the five lowest and largest bones of the spinal column. Most of the body's weight and stress falls on the lumbar vertebrae. Below the lumbar region is the sacrum, a shield-shaped bony structure that connects with the pelvis at the sacroiliac joints. At the end of the sacrum are two to four tiny partially fused vertebrae known as the coccyx or "tail bone."

Vertebrae in the spinal column are separated from each other by small cushions of cartilage known as intervertebral discs. Inside each disc is a jelly-like substance called the nucleus pulposus, which is surrounded by a fibrous structure. The disc is 80% water, which makes it very elastic. It has no blood supply of its own, however, but relies on nearby blood vessels to keep it nourished.

Each vertebra in the spine has a number of bony projections, known as processes. The spinal and transverse processes attach to the muscles in the back and act like little levers, allowing the spine to twist or bend.

The articular processes from the joints between the vertebrae themselves, meeting together and interlocking at the facet joints. Each vertebra and its processes surround and protect an arch-shaped central opening. These arches, aligned to run down the spine, form the spinal canal, which encloses the spinal cord, the central trunk of nerves that connects the brain with the rest of the body. Each nerve root passes from the spinal column to other parts of the body through small openings bounded on one side by the disc and the other by the facets. When the spinal cord reaches the lumbar region, it splits into four bundled strands of nerve roots called the cauda equina (meaning horsetail in Latin).

Viewed laterally the vertebral column presents several curves, which correspond to the different regions of the column, and are called cervical, thoracic, lumbar, and pelvic.

The cervical curve, convex forward, begins at the apex of the odontoid (*tooth-like*) process, and ends at the middle of the second thoracic vertebra; it is the least marked of all the curves.

The thoracic curve, concave forward, begins at the middle of the second and ends at the middle of the twelfth thoracic vertebra. Its most prominent point behind corresponds to the spinous process of the seventh thoracic vertebra. This curve is known as a *tt curve.*

The lumbar curve is more marked in the female than in the male; it begins at the middle of the last thoracic vertebra, and ends at the sacrovertebral angle. It is convex anteriorly, the convexity of the lower three vertebrae being much greater than that of the upper two. This curve is described as a *lordotic curve.*

The pelvic curve begins at the sacrovertebral articulation, and ends at the point of the coccyx; its concavity is directed downward and forward.

The thoracic and pelvic curves are termed **primary curves**, because they alone are present during fetal life. The cervical and lumbar curves are *compensatory* or *secondary*, and are developed after birth, the former when the child is able to hold up its head (at three or four months) and to sit upright (at nine months), and the latter at twelve or eighteen months, when the child begins to walk.

The spinal column (or vertebral column) extends from the skull to the pelvis and is made up of 33 individual bones termed vertebrae. The vertebrae are stacked on top of each other group into four regions:

Cervical Vertebrae (C1 – C7)

The seven "cervical vertebrae" comprise the bony axis of the neck. Although these are the smallest of the vertebrae, their bone tissues are denser than those in any other region of the column. The transverse processes of the cervical vertebrae are distinctive because they have "transverse foramina", which serve as passageways for arteries leading to the brain. Also, the "spinous processes" of the second through the fifth cervical vertebrae are uniquely forked. These processes provide attachments for various muscles. Two of the cervical vertebrae are of special interest. The first vertebra ("atlas") supports and balances the head. It has practically no body or spine and appears as a bony ring with two transverse processes. On its upper surface, the atlas has two kidney-shaped facets that unite with the occipital condyles of the skull. The second vertebra is the "axis," which bears a tooth-like "odontoid process" on its body. This process projects upward and lies in the ring of the atlas. As the head is turned from side to side, the atlas pivots around the odontoid process.

The cervical spine is further divided into two parts; the upper cervical region (C_1 and C_2), and the lower cervical region (C_3 through C_7). C_1 is termed the Atlas and C_2 the Axis. The **Occiput** (CO), also known as the Occipital Bone, is a flat bone that forms the back of the head.

Atlas (C1)

The Atlas is the first cervical vertebra and therefore abbreviated C_1. This vertebra supports the skull. Its appearance is different from the other spinal vertebrae. The atlas is a ring of bone made up of two lateral masses joined at the front and back by the anterior arch and the posterior arch.

Axis (C2)

The Axis is the second cervical vertebra or C_2. It is a blunt tooth–like process that projects upward. It is also referred to as the 'dens' (Latin for 'tooth') or odontoid process. The dens provides a type of pivot and collar allowing the head and atlas to rotate around the dens.

Thoracic Vertebrae (T1 – T12)

The thoracic vertebrae increase in size from T1 through T12. They are characterized by small pedicles, long spinous processes, and relatively large intervertebral foramen (neural passageways), which result in less incidence of nerve compression.

The rib cage is joined to the thoracic vertebrae. At T11 and T12, the ribs do not attach and are so are called "floating ribs." The thoracic spine's range of motion is limited due to the many rib/vertebrae connections and the long spinous processes

Lumbar Vertebrae (L1 – L5)

The lumbar vertebrae graduate in size from L1 through L5. These vertebrae bear much of the body's weight and related biomechanical stress. The pedicles are longer and wider than those in the thoracic spine. The spinous processes are horizontal and more squared in shape. The intervertebral foramen (neural passageways) are relatively large but nerve root compression is more common than in the thoracic spine.

Sacral Spine

The Sacrum is located behind the pelvis. Five bones (abbreviated S1 through S5) fused into a triangular shape, form the sacrum. The sacrum fits between the two hipbones connecting the spine to the pelvis. The last lumbar vertebra (L5) articulates (moves) with the sacrum. Immediately below the sacrum are five additional bones, fused together to form the Coccyx (tailbone).

The Coccyx

The coccyx (or tail) is the lowest part of the vertebral column and is attached by ligaments to the margins of the sacral hiatus. When a person is sitting, pressure is exerted on the coccyx, and it moves forward, acting sort of like a shock absorber. Sitting down with too great a force may cause the coccyx to be fractured or dislocated.

Purpose of the Vertebrae

Although vertebrae range in size; cervical the smallest, lumbar the largest, vertebral bodies are the weight bearing structures of the spinal column. Upper body weight is distributed through the spine to the sacrum and pelvis. The natural curves in the spine, kyphotic and lordotic, provide resistance and elasticity in distributing body weight and axial loads sustained during movement.

The vertebrae are composed of many elements that are critical to the overall function of the spine, which include the intervertebral discs and facet joints.

Functions of the Vertebral or Spinal Column Include:

Protection	■ Spinal Cord and Nerve Roots ■ Many internal organs
Base for Attachment	■ Ligaments ■ Tendons ■ Muscles
Structural Support	■ Head, shoulders, chest ■ Connects upper and lower body ■ Balance and weight distribution
Flexibility and Mobility	■ Flexion (forward bending) ■ Extension (backward bending) ■ Side bending (left and right) ■ Rotation (left and right) ■ Combination of above
Other	■ Bones produce red blood cells ■ Mineral storage

Aside from the functions listed above, the spinal cord regulates some important unconscious (or automatic) body functions, including bowel and bladder control, and normal sexual organ function. These controls are governed by the lowest part of the cord, called the conus medullaris, and are transmitted by the sacral nerve roots.

The cord is composed of an outer layer of white matter and a central area of gray matter. In the white matter are major fiber tracts. These bundles of nerves carry messages up (sensory information) and down (motor commands) the spinal cord, to and from the brain. There are many more fiber tracts than are shown, many involving control of unconscious functions.

Connections between nerve cells are located in the gray matter. These connections, like the circuit boards in computers, process information received and sends out commands in response. Trillions of nerve fibers are involved, the complexity in the spinal cord alone is far greater than any man-made computer yet conceived.

This naturally leads us to consider another vital part of human anatomy; the nervous system.

Nerves (key to whole body)

Nerve tissue

Nerve tissues carry information to and from the brain to control how the body works. There are two major divisions of nerve tissue: the central nervous system (called the CNS) composed of the brain and spinal cord, and the peripheral nervous system (or PNS) composed of the nerves and nerve endings in the rest of the body. The CNS functions much like a computer. It receives messages from many areas of the body and sends out commands in response. Information and messages are processed in some parts of the brain consciously (thinking), and in other parts of the brain and in the spinal cord unconsciously (reflex response). The PNS does not process information, but only transmits messages back and forth between the CNS and the rest of the body.

Nerves control the body's functions including the vital organs, sensation, and movement. The nervous system receives information and initiates an appropriate response. It is affected by internal and external factors (i.e. stimuli).

Nerves follow tracts and cross over junctions called synapses. Simplified, it is a complex communicative process between nerves conducted by chemical and/or electrical changes.

The skin of the body can be mapped out into separate areas called dermatomes. Each dermatome is supplied by a separate nerve root. By testing for sensation (feeling) in a specific dermatome, it is possible to find out whether that dermatome's nerve root is connected to the conscious portion of the brain.

Motor function carried by the nerve roots can be tested. It is well known which nerve roots provide control to which muscles. In this manner, nerve root function is easily tested.

Central Nervous System (CNS)

The Central Nervous System is composed of the brain and spinal cord. The brain has 12 cranial nerves. The spinal cord, which originates immediately below the brain stem, extends to the first lumbar vertebra (L1). Beyond L1 the spinal cord becomes the cauda equina. The spinal cord provides a means of communication between the brain and peripheral nerves.

BRAIN	12 Cranial Nerves
Motor:	5 nerves
Sensory:	3 Nerves
Motor/Sensory:	4 nerves
SPINAL CORD	31 Pairs – Spinal Nerves
Cervical	8 pair
Thoracic	12 pair
Lumbar	5 pair
Sacral	5 pair
Coccyx	1 pair

Peripheral Nervous System (PNS)

The CNS extends to the Peripheral Nervous System, a system of nerves that branch beyond the spinal cord, brain, and brain-stem. The PNS carries information to and from the CNS.

The PNS includes the **Somatic Nervous System (SNS)** and the **Autonomic Nervous System (ANS)**. The somatic nervous system includes the nerves serving the musculoskeletal system and the skin. It is voluntary and reacts to outside stimuli affecting the body. The autonomic nervous system is involuntary automatically seeking to maintain homeostasis or normal function.

The ANS is further divided into the **Sympathetic Nervous System** and the **Parasympathetic Nervous System.** The sympathetic nervous system is an involuntary system often associated with the flight or fight response. The parasympathetic nervous system is responsible for promoting internal harmony such as regular heartbeat during normal activity.

Just below the last thoracic (T12) and first lumbar (L1) vertebra the spinal cord ends at the **Conus Medullaris**. From this point the spinal nerves, resembling a horse's tail become known as the **cauda equina** extending to the coccyx. These nerves are suspended in spinal fluid.

Spinal Nerves	
Motor	• Anterior Roots • Ventral Roots
Sensory	• Posterior Roots • Dorsal Roots

Other Spinal Cord and Nerve Structures

Cerebrospinal Fluid (CSF)

Cerebrospinal fluid is a clear fluid found in the brain chambers (Ventricles), spinal canal, and spinal cord. This fluid is secreted from the Choroids Plexus, a vascular part in the ventricles of the brain. CSF bathes and circulates among these tissues and acts as a shock absorber to protect against injury. The fluid contains different electrolytes, proteins, and glucose. In an average adult the total volume of CSF is about 150 millilitres.

Meninges

Meninges are membranes that cover and protect the brain and spinal cord. There are three primary types: (1) Dura Mater, (2) Arachnoid Mater, and (3) Pia Mater.

1. The dura mater, or dura, is the gray outer layer of the spinal cord and nerve roots. It is made of strong connective tissue.

2. The arachnoid mater resembles a loosely woven fabric of arteries and veins. This layer is thinner than the dura mater. The Subarachnoid space is filled with cerebrospinal fluid.

3. The pia mater is the innermost layer and is a delicate and highly vascular membrane providing blood to the neural structures.

Dermatomes

A dermatome is an area of skin supplied by fibers from a single spinal nerve root.

Ligaments and tendons

Ligaments and tendons are soft collagenous tissues. Ligaments connect bone to bone and tendons connect muscles to bone. Ligaments and tendons play a significant role in musculoskeletal biomechanics. They represent an important area of orthopaedic treatment for which many challenges for repair remain.

Most of these challenges have to do with restoring the normal mechanical function of these tissues. Again, as with all biological tissues, ligaments and tendons have a hierarchical structure that affects their mechanical behaviour. In addition, ligaments and tendons can adapt to changes in their mechanical environment due to injury, disease or exercise. Thus, ligaments and tendons are another example of the structure-function concept and the mechanically mediated adaptation concept that permeate this biomechanics course. In this section, we will review aspects of ligament and tendon structure, function and adaptation.

The ligament or tendon then is split into smaller entities called fascicles. The fascicle contains the basic fibril of the ligament or tendon, and the fibroblasts, which are the biological cells that produce the ligament or tendon. There is a structural characteristic at this level that plays a significant role in the mechanics of ligaments and tendons: the crimp of the fibril. The crimp is the waviness of the fibril; we will see that this contributes significantly to the nonlinear stress strain relationship for ligaments and tendons and indeed for basically all soft collagenous tissues.

People often talk about tendons and ligaments as if they are the same thing, but these two types of soft tissue actually perform different functions for the body.

Tendons

A tendon connects muscle to bone. These tough, yet flexible, bands of fibrous tissue attach to the skeletal muscles that move your bones. Tendons essentially enable one to move since they act as intermediaries between the muscles creating the motion of the bones.

I'd say the most famous tendon is the Achilles tendon (named after a Greek Mythology character) which connects the muscles of your calf to your heel. Also, if you watch the tops of your hands while you type, you can see your tendons at work.

Anatomy:

1. Tendons contain collagen fibrils (Type 1)

2. Tendons contain a proteoglycan matrix

3. Tendons contain fibroblasts (biological cells) that are arranged in parallel rows

Basic Functions

1. Tendons carry tensite forces from muscle to bone

2. Tendons carry compressive forces when wrapped around bone like a pulley

Ligaments

Ligaments are fibrous bands or sheets of connective tissue linking two or more bones, cartilages, or structures together. One or more ligaments provide stability to a joint during rest and movement. Excessive movements such as hyper–extension or hyper–flexion may be restricted by ligaments. Further, some ligaments prevent movement in certain directions.

Ligaments are similar to tendons, but they connect bone to bone and help to stabilize joints. They are composed mostly of long, stringy collagen fibers creating short bands of tough fibrous connective tissue.

Ligaments are slightly elastic, so they can be stretched to gradually lengthen increasing flexibility. Athletes and dancers stretch their ligaments to make their joints more supple, and to prevent injury.

The term double-jointed refers to people who have more elastic ligaments.

You might have heard of some of the ligaments found in the knee since they often tear, especially the ACL (Anterior Cruciate Ligament) when skiing. In fact four ligaments connect the tibia (shin bone) to the femur (thigh bone) to provide structure for the knee.

Anatomy

1. Similar to the tendon in hierarchical structure

2. Collagen fibrils are slightly less in volume fraction and organization than in a tendon.

3. Higher percentage of proteoglycan matrix than tendons

4. Fibroblasts

Blood Supply

1. Microvascularity from insertion site

2. Nutrition for cell population; necessary synthesis and repair

Three of the more important ligaments in the spine are the Ligamentum Flavum, Anterior Longitudinal Ligament and the Posterior Longitudinal Ligament.

- The Ligamentum Flavum forms a cover over the dura mater: a layer of tissue that protects the spinal cord. This ligament connects under the facet joints to create a small curtain over the posterior openings between the vertebrae.

- The Anterior Longitudinal Ligament attaches to the front (anterior) of each vertebra. This ligament runs up and down the spine (vertical or longitudinal).

- The Posterior Longitudinal Ligament runs up and down behind (posterior) the spine and **Ligament Systems – Atlas and Axis**.

As mentioned in the Vertebral Column, the Atlas (C1) and Axis (C2) are different from the other spinal vertebrae. The upper cervical ligament system is especially important in stabilizing the upper cervical spine from the skull to C2. Although the cervical vertebrae are the smallest, the neck has the greatest range of motion.

Occipitoatlantal Ligament Complex (Atlas)

These three ligaments run between the Occiput and the Atlas:

- Anterior Occipitoatlantal Ligament
- Posterior Occipitoatlantal Ligament
- Lateral Occipitoatlantal Ligaments (2)

Occipitioaxial Ligament Complex (Axis)

These three ligaments connect the Occiput to the Axis:

- Occipitoaxial Ligament
- Alar Ligaments (2)
- Apical Ligament

Altantoxial Ligament Complex (Axis)

These three ligaments extend from the Atlas to the Axis:

- Anterior Atlantoaxial Ligament
- Posterior Atlantoaxial Ligament
- Lateral Ligaments (2)

Cruciate Ligament Complex

These ligaments help to stabilize the Atlantoaxial (Axis) complex:

- Transverse Ligaments
- Superior Longitudinal Fascicles
- Inferior Longitudinal Fascicles
- inside the spinal canal.

CHAPTER 3

Chiropractic 101

HERE'S HOW SIGNIFICANT your nerves and therefore the chiropractic profession is. Consider that a normal human being can live up to 6 weeks without food, 6 days without water, 6 minutes without a heart and only 6 milliseconds without nerves.

A doctor of chiropractic (DC), chiropractor or chiropractic physician is a medical professional who is trained to diagnose and treat disorders of the musculoskeletal and nervous systems. Chiropractors treat patients of all ages—infants, children, and adults. They believe in a conservative (non-surgical) hands-on approach to treating these disorders.

The understanding that the spine is involved in health and wellness, as well as the practice of using manual manipulation as a source of healing, dates back to the time of the ancient Greek philosophers. In fact, Hippocrates once said, "Get knowledge of the spine, for this is the requisite for many diseases."

Modern chiropractic, however, marks its beginnings in the late 1800s, when a Canadian living in the US, Daniel David Palmer, a self-educated teacher and healer, performed the first spinal manipulation on a patient.

That patient was Harvey Lillard, a janitor who worked in Palmer's building. Lillard was nearly totally deaf and mentioned to Palmer that he lost his hearing many years before when he was bending over and felt a "pop" in his upper back.

Palmer, who was a practitioner of magnet therapy (a common therapy of the time), was quite knowledgeable in anatomy and very interested in how the spine interacts with the rest of the body's systems. He felt strongly that the two events—the "popping" in Lillard's back and his deafness—must somehow be related.

He examined Lillard's spine and found a problem with one of his vertebra. Palmer manipulated Lillard's vertebra and an amazing event occurred—Lillard's hearing was restored. Today, this procedure is known as a chiropractic adjustment.

Palmer soon discovered that adjustments could relieve patients' pain and other symptoms. These problems with vertebrae have been called chiropractic subluxations.

He began to use these "hand treatments" to treat a variety of ailments, including sciatica, migraine headaches, stomach complaints, epilepsy, and heart trouble. In 1898, he opened the Palmer School & Infirmary of Chiropractic in Davenport, Iowa, and began teaching his chiropractic techniques to others.

The medical community did not immediately embrace Palmer's chiropractic theories and techniques. They called him a "quack" and refused to acknowledge his accomplishments. At one point, Palmer was even indicted for practicing medicine without a license and spent time in jail for his offense.

Research has shown that Palmer was not the ignorant "fish monger" that some in the medical profession claim. An investigation of particular libraries, which he quoted from liberally in his letters, showed that he was up to date in his knowledge at the turn of the 20th century.

Current Research

Many studies have recently shown that chiropractic care is cost-effective, safe and helpful for patients. Recent studies have shown that chiropractic patients have three times the satisfaction rate of medical patients. The National Institute of Health performed a full study of all types of treatments for lower back pain, including medications, physical therapy, acupuncture, and chiropractic, and found that chiropractic care was the most effective type of treatment for lower back pain. This study was later confirmed by Consumer Reports. Another study performed evaluated the cost effectiveness of chiropractic care. This study found that the average chiropractic user saved 1,500 dollars by going to a chiropractor for their care. A large study by Duke University evaluated all the treatment types available for cervicogenic or tension type headaches. This study evaluated prescription and over the counter medications, as well as physical therapy and acupuncture. This study once again showed that chiropractic care was the most effective type of treatment for these types of headaches. In addition, recent studies show that chiropractic is the most utilized alternative healthcare in the United States.

Chiropractic Today

Today, chiropractors are licensed in all the US states, Canadian provinces, most European countries, Australia and New Zealand. There are more than 50,000 practicing chiropractors in the US alone. In addition, despite its North American roots, there are now more chiropractic educational programs outside of North America than there are in North America. Chiropractic continues to gain wide acceptance by the medical, legal, and patient communities through its record of beneficial results and ongoing research

A visit with a doctor of chiropractic is similar to other doctor appointments. The chiropractor takes the patient's medical history, performs a physical and orthopedic neurological examination, and relies on other tests, such as diagnostic imaging and blood tests.

After a diagnosis is made, the chiropractor recommends a treatment plan. If the patient's disorder is beyond the scope of chiropractic care, the doctor refers the patient to the appropriate healthcare provider. Many times chiropractors co-treat patients with other healthcare providers.

Chiropractors do not perform surgery. Although hands-on manipulation of the problem-specific joints is central to chiropractic, treatment focuses on whole-body health. Working toward restoring and maintaining overall health may include physiological therapeutics and lifestyle counseling.

Chiropractic education is a very rigorous and strenuous undertaking. Before entering an accredited chiropractic school, a potential student must first complete a Bachelor of Science degree from an accredited institution, focusing on biology, chemistry and anatomy. After a four year degree, a student may then apply to a chiropractic college. Screening process for entering chiropractic care is very thorough and includes transcripts, grades, testing, and a thorough interview process. Upon acceptance to a chiropractic college, a student then enrolls in a three semester a year program lasting three and a half years of book study. Students take an average of 25 credits per trimester or 75-85 credits per year for almost four years. In addition to the classroom hours, three national board exams, consisting of three days of monitored testing, must be completed. Upon completion of these hours, a final year of clinical experience is warranted in which a student continues classroom learning, but spends 10 hours a day in a clinic, treating patients, performing x-rays and other evaluations. Upon completion of their requisites a student may then sit for the fourth part of the National Boards and once they pass they will receive their degree. After all this testing, the final hurdle is a state licensing test in order for the applicant to work in the state they choose.

Chiropractors treat many musculoskeletal and nervous system disorders and conditions that affect the spine. Many are listed below.

- Back sprain or strain
- Coccydynia (tailbone pain)
- Degenerative disc disease
- Myofascial pain/trigger points
- Fibromyalgia
- Headaches (certain types)
- Herniated and bulging discs

- Piriformis syndrome
- Sciatica
- Spondylosis (osteoarthritis)
- Whiplash
- Scoliosis
- Short leg syndrome
- Sports injuries
- Upper back pain
- Peripheral neuropathies
- Tendinitis/tendinosis

CHAPTER 4

Stress 101
Managing Stress:

WHEN ONE IS IN PAIN or under any stress, muscles contract, which causes more pain. The muscles in the back and neck are especially sensitive to stress. Stress hormones that are released when one is under stress increase the perception of pain and may trigger depression, which is common with fibromyalgia.

The Stress / Back Pain Connection

There is a strong connection between stress and back pain. Stress causes a release of stress hormones. Stress hormones increase the perception of pain.

Stress hormones also cause the muscles to tighten up. The muscles may tense up so much they go into painful spasms. Back and neck muscles are particularly sensitive to the effects of stress.

Muscle tension reduces blood flow to the tissues (reduced oxygen and nutrients to the tissues). Reduced blood flow delays healing. Adequate circulation is also necessary to flush acidic waste products (byproducts of muscular activity) from the tissues. A build up of acidic waste products in the tissues can cause fatigue and pain.

Stress in itself can cause back pain. A person with a 'bad back', for example, a person who has scar tissue from an old injury or degenerative changes in the spine due to aging, may notice the effects of stress triggering back pain even more than someone with a healthy back. The slightest muscle tension may be 'the straw the broke the camel's back.' For instance, if spinal nerves are already restricted by scar tissue or calcium deposits, it may take minimal muscle tension to compress nerves and cause pain. Sciatica may flare up when one is feeling stressed.

Tense back muscles increase back pain and pain increases tensing of muscles – *and a vicious cycle of stress and back pain can be created.*

The back is less capable of tolerating even mild abuse (lifting something slightly heavy, poor posture, a sudden twist, sitting too long, etc) when a person is under stress. Stress causes the muscles to tighten up, leaving them vulnerable to injury.

Types of Stress

Everyone realizes how mental stress can affect the body, as nearly everyone has had a bad day at work and felt tension in the neck muscles. However this type of common stress is just one type of stress the body deals with. There are three distinct types of stress that affect the human body:

Chemical Stress

Two things cause chemical stress: number one, not enough proper nutrients and nutrition feeding the body, causing it to undergo stress and break down. The second is having improper chemicals being put into the body. This includes things such as medications, alcohol, improper diet, non-prescription medications, and bad nutrients.

Emotional Stress

Having a traumatic incident in one's life not only affects the mental state but the physical state of the person as well. Everyone has heard of a situation in which a couple has been married 50 years; one spouse gets ill and passes, and the second seemingly healthy spouse gets sick and passes a few months later. This is not coincidence; this is due to the emotional trauma affecting the immune system and general well being of the body

Physical Stress

Physical stress is what we commonly think of as injuries to the body. This includes things like a trip and fall, car accident, sports injury, or any way in which the body is physically damaged. These are the injuries people most commonly think about, but represent just a portion of all the stress our bodies undergo.

Reducing Stress

Relieving stress can reduce pain that is aggravated or caused by tense muscles. Managing stress on an ongoing basis may also help prevent back pain from occurring in the first place.

Exercise

Stress can be relieved through exercise. Aerobic exercise is a particularly effective form of exercise for relieving stress. This is because aerobic exercise burns off stress hormones and increases the body's production of endorphins, which are naturally occurring chemicals that relieve pain and improve mood. Stretching exercises also can relieve stress and loosen tight muscles. Yoga incorporates poses that increase strength and flexibility with breathing techniques to relieve stress.

Relaxation Techniques

Relaxation techniques invoke the "relaxation response." Muscles relax and blood pressure, heartbeat, and respiration decrease. This is the opposite of the "stress response" where muscles tense and blood pressure, heartbeat, and respiration increase.

There are many relaxation techniques, from simple deep breathing exercises that are easy to learn on one's own to self-hypnosis that must initially be taught by a qualified professional. Other relaxation techniques include meditation, progressive muscle relaxation, guided imagery and biofeedback.

Though most relaxation techniques are not complicated, they still take time and practice to master.

Common Back Problems, Brief explanation

Disc bulge

The intervertebral discs are the spongy cushions between the vertebrae. As we age, these discs dry out and harden, making them prone to injury. The disc doesn't actually move out of place, but can bulge (prolapse). This is called a 'disc bulge'.

Studies are finding that bulging and protruding discs show up on the scans of up to 60% of people who have no back pain at all. Experts now generally believe that bulging, or even protruding, discs may be normal and do not necessarily indicate serious back problems. One expert suggested that discs might even swell in response to stress and then contract again. However, disc material that extrudes (that is, it balloons into the area outside the vertebrae or breaks off from the disc) will most likely cause pain. Sciatic pain is also sometimes present when there is no bulging or extruding of the discs. Most disc bulges can be treated conservatively; chiropractic care is great at relieving pain and pressure from a disc bulge and can be combined with ultrasound, muscle traction, or other techniques to alleviate your pain. More severe disc bulges may be treated with non-surgical spinal decompression. This treatment will be discussed later in the book, however, using précised computer controlled decompression can allow the disc to rehydrate and also pull back into its original position. Which will allow normal function of the disc, not just temporarily alleviating the symptoms. Medical management of disc bulges often consists of steroid injections, pain medication, and sometimes surgical intervention.

Disc Herniation

A herniated disc, sometimes (but incorrectly) called a slipped disc, is the most common cause of severe sciatica. A disc in the lumbar area becomes herniated when it ruptures or when the gelatin within the disc protrudes outward. If the material breaks off or extends far enough out to press against the nerve root, sciatic pain can occur. Some cases of chronic low back pain may be caused by inward growth of nerve fibers into intervertebral discs. Some evidence also exists that nerves in the outer ring of the disc may be the source of pain.

Most disc problems arise from prolonged stress or injury and may be caused by straining the back (such as when lifting).

Most disc herniations can also be treated conservatively with chiropractic care, ultrasound, muscle traction, laser, etc. Some, however, are too large or put too much pressure on the nerves and may need epidural injections, decompression surgery, or even more invasive procedures. However the vast majority can be treated with conservative care, including non surgical spinal decompression, MUA, ultrasound, chiropractic, and more.

Pinched nerves,

Nerves Carry Signals Throughout the Body

A peripheral nerve is like a fiber-optic cable, with many fibers encased in an outer sheath. You can think of each individual fiber as a microscopic garden hose. The green part of the hose is a fine membrane where a static electrical charge can travel to or from the brain. The inside of the hose transports fluid from the nerve cell body that helps nourish and replenish the ever-changing components of the green part, or membrane.

If the nerve is pinched, the flow up and down the inside of the hose is reduced or blocked, meaning nutrients stop flowing. Eventually, the membrane starts to lose its healthy ability to transmit tiny electrical charges and the nerve fiber may eventually die. When enough fibers stop working, a muscle may not contract and skin may feel numb.

Causes of a Pinched Nerve

A nerve can be pinched as it leaves the spine by a herniated disc or bone spurs that form from spinal arthritis. Another commonplace for pinched nerves is the carpal tunnel. This is a bottleneck area, through which all the finger flexor tendons and the median nerve must pass to the hand. Regardless of where the nerve is pinched, in the neck or carpal tunnel, the patient often will feel similar symptoms of numbness in the hand, because the brain does not know how to tell the difference between the beginning, middle, or end of a nerve. It only knows that it is not receiving signals from the hand, and so numbness begins.

Symptoms of a Pinched Nerve

A pinched nerve in the low back usually is perceived as radiating down the leg. Here again, the symptoms the person experiences seem to be traveling into the leg along the usual path. This is the basis of *referred pain*.

Muscle spasm in the back commonly accompanies pinched nerves and can be quite painful.

Sometimes, nerves can be pinched and the only symptoms may be numbness and weakness in the arm or leg *without* pain. Other symptoms include tingling, burning, electric, and a hot/cold sensation.

Pinched nerves and chiropractic care go hand in hand. Whether the nerve is pinched in the spine as is most common, or in an arm, leg, or anywhere, pinched nerves respond perfectly to conservative chiropractic care, and therapies if needed.

Arthritis

There are many types of back and neck disorders that affect the majority of the population in the United States. Injury, aging, general health, and lifestyle may influence the development of some conditions. Most spinal disorders are known to result from soft tissue injury, structural injury, and degenerative or congenital conditions.

At birth the structural integrity of the spine, heart, lungs, and other organ systems is at its peak for future development. During mid-life early microscopic changes begin to appear that indicate the spine is aging. The spine does not deteriorate just because of age. Wear and tear is also responsible. Disorders such as arthritis, spinal stenosis, and osteoporosis do not develop overnight. Degenerative diseases may take years to develop and may be associated with past injury, abuse, body structure, or congenital problems.

Millions of people suffer from arthritis. In fact, arthritis affects approximately 80% of people over the age of 55 in the United States. It is estimated that by the year 2020, over 60 million people will suffer from this often-disabling problem.

Arthritis may affect the joints in the spine, which enable the body to bend and twist. Part of the problem may be the body's response to arthritis, which is to manufacture extra bone to stop joint movement. The extra bone is called a bone spur or bony overgrowth.

In medical terms, the extra bone is called an osteophyte. **Osteophytes** may be found in areas affected by arthritis such as the disc or joint spaces where cartilage has deteriorated. The body's production of osteophytes is a futile attempt to stop the motion of the arthritic joint and deal with the degenerative process. It never completely works. The evidence of bony deposits can be found on an x-ray. A bone spur may cause nerve impingement at the neuroforamen. The neuroforamen are passageways through which the nerve roots exit the spinal canal. Sensory symptoms include pain, numbness, burning and pins and needles in the extremities below the affected spinal nerve root. Motor symptoms include muscle spasm, cramping, weakness, or loss of muscular control in a part of the body.

Arthritis is actually a term for over 100 rheumatoid disorders. Common forms include:

- Osteoarthritis
- Rheumatoid Arthritis
- Ankylosing Spondylitis
- Juvenile Arthritis
- Psoriatic Arthritis
- Systemic Lupus Erythematosus

Arthritis can affect any part of the body, even the spine.

Inflammatory arthritis is an autoimmune disease. Autoimmune disorders cause the body to mistakenly attack its own immune system. Normally, the immune's systems B and T cells work together to find, attack and destroy foreign substances, such as a virus or toxin. Evidence of antibody production is found in the blood.

In people with healthy a healthy immune system, the body produces antibodies that help fight disease and illness. However, in patients with inflammatory arthritis, antibodies attack the joints and ligaments, including those in the spine.

Inflammatory arthritis is set apart from osteoarthritis, the more common form of joint degeneration.

For reasons not completely understood, rheumatoid arthritis (RA) usually affects the cervical (neck) spine. Rarely is the disease found in the thoracolumbar (mid and low back) regions. It is more common in adult women and is characterized by 2 or more swollen and inflamed joints. Neck symptoms may include headache, neck pain, numbness, tingling, and weakness in the arms and legs

Any doctor who tells you that they can cure your arthritis is clearly lying to you. However, arthritis can be treated conservatively and symptom relief is usually easily obtained. Chiropractic care in addition to therapies can alleviate the pain in most cases, and natural herbal and nutritional methods can be used to decrease swelling and improve flexibility. These procedures when combined with exercise, diet modification, and healthy lifestyle can ensure years of good relief. However, the underlying arthritis will always be there.

Spinal Stenosis

Spinal Stenosis is a type of arthritis of the spine. It most commonly affects the lumbar spine, the lower back, but it can also effect the cervical spine or neck. This type of degeneration of the spine occurs when the central canal begins narrowing. This can happen due to age or can be an inherited or congenital problem. The central canal of the spine is the middle opening of the bones which holds the spinal canal, which is the tree trunk of the nervous system. The spinal cord has the branches of the cord, which are the spinal nerves, that control all the cells tissues and organs. The spinal cord is a direct link from the brain, which transfers all nerve activity to the spinal nerves and the rest of the tissues. The narrowing of the canal doesn't allow nerve signal to get to the correct body parts. Usually this occurs in the lower back, which doesn't allow the brain to talk to the legs. This can induce leg pain, weakness, numbness in the legs, and trouble walking. Usually this is aggravated by standing and walking. Stenosis can be a serious medical problem. Severe cases may require surgery, as severe stenosis can inhibit the nerve signals to the bowel and bladder and cause problems urinated and defecating. Moderate to mild cases can be treated with spinal decompression, which will be discussed later in the book.

Tendinitis

Tendinitis Causes

The most common cause of tendinitis is overuse and repetitive motion from recreational, athletic, or occupational activities. Risk factors for tendonitis include repetitive movement, trauma, thermal injury to the tendon, use of certain antibiotics (such as levofloxacin and ciprofloxacin), and smoking. Tendinitis can also occur in people with diseases such as rheumatoid arthritis, obesity, and diabetes.

These are some of the more common forms of tendinitis:

- Medial epicondylitis (golfer's elbow, baseball elbow, suitcase elbow) is caused by inflammation of the tendons that attach to the medial epicondyle of the elbow. If you put your arms to your side with the palms facing forward, the medial epicondyle is the bony part of the elbow nearest to your body. Repetitive movements involving forceful wrist flexion and rotation can cause this elbow tendinitis.

- Lateral epicondylitis (tennis elbow) is caused by inflammation of the tendons that attach to the lateral epicondyle of the elbow. If you put your arms to your side with the palms facing forward, the lateral epicondyle is the bony part of the elbow farthest away from your body. Repetitive movements involving extension and rotation of the wrist can cause this elbow tendinitis.

- Rotator cuff tendinitis (swimmer's shoulder, tennis shoulder, pitcher's shoulder) is caused by sports that require movement of the arm over the head repeatedly. This repetitive motion causes inflammation on the rotator cuff, a group of muscles that control shoulder rotation. The supraspinatus, infraspinatus, teres minor, and subscapularis tendons form the rotator cuff tendons.

- Calcific tendinitis is caused by calcium deposits in the rotator cuff tendons.

- Bicipital tendinitis is inflammation of the tendon that attaches the biceps muscle (located in the front of the arm) to the shoulder. Wear and tear over time or overuse are common causes of bicipital tendinitis.

- Patellar tendinitis (jumper's knee) is inflammation of the patellar tendon that attaches the kneecap to the tibia. Patellar tendinitis is caused by repetitive jumping, running, or cutting movements.

- Popliteus tendinitis is a form of tendinitis behind the knee caused by downhill running or walking.

- Achilles tendinitis is caused by downhill running, jumping, or other activities that can strain the calf muscles.

- Peroneal tendinitis is inflammation of the tendon that is located in the side of the ankle and foot. Excessive hiking, tennis, or many other activities may cause peroneal tendinitis.

- De Quervain's tenosynovitis is a painful inflammation of the tendons on the thumb side of the wrist. De Quervain's tenosynovitis is caused by repetitive movements of the wrist and hand, such as lifting up young children from under their armpits.

- Most if not all tendinits cases respond well to conservative care using muscle stimulation, cold laser therapy, and stretching done by a qualified doctor of chiropractic.

Sprain vs. strain

An out-of-condition back or one with pre-existing problems is more susceptible to soft tissue injuries like sprains and strains.

- **Sprain** – a joint injury that involves stretching or tearing of the ligaments.
- **Strain** – an injury to muscle or tendons.

Stretching a ligament or muscle too far or too quickly could result in a tear of the tissue. Excessive force and repetitive use may also damage muscles. Most sprain/ strain injuries will slowly heal on their own. To speed up the process or for more advanced cases, these soft-tissue injuries can be treated well with ultrasound, EMS stimulation, stretching and other conservative measures done by your chiropractor.

Chiropractic subluxation

The WHO definition of the chiropractic vertebral subluxation is:

"A lesion or dysfunction in a joint or motion segment in which alignment, movement integrity and/or physiological function are altered, although contact between joint surfaces remains intact. It is essentially a functional entity, which may influence biomechanical and neural integrity."

The purported displacement is not necessarily visible on X-rays. This is in contrast to the medical definition of spinal subluxation which, according to the WHO, is a *"significant structural displacement"*, and therefore visible on X-rays.

In 1996 an official consensus definition of subluxation was formed. Cooperstein and Gleberzon have described the situation: "... although many in the chiropractic profession reject the concept of "subluxation" and shun the use of this term as a diagnosis, the presidents of at least a dozen chiropractic colleges of the Association of Chiropractic Colleges developed a consensus definition of "subluxation" in 1996. It reads:

> "Chiropractic is concerned with the preservation and restoration of health, and focuses particular attention on the subluxation. A subluxation is a complex of functional and/or structural and/or pathological articular changes that compromise neural integrity and may influence organ system function and general health. A subluxation is evaluated, diagnosed, and managed through the use of chiropractic procedures based on the best available rational and empirical evidence."

Chiropractors believe that good health is determined by a healthy nervous system, particularly a healthy spinal column. Occasionally, vertebrae become misaligned and place pressure on the nerves exiting the spinal cord. The misalignment of a vertebra is called a chiropractic subluxation.

Chiropractic is based on the theory that if the spinal column is properly aligned, nerve impulses can freely flow along the spinal cord. If the spinal column is out of alignment (a subluxation), the flow of nerve impulses is interrupted and disease (not just back pain) result. This is called the subluxation theory. According to the subluxation theory, disorders in any area of the body can result from subluxations in the spine as the nervous system carries messages to all areas of the body. Restoring the vertebrae to proper alignment restores proper functioning of the nervous system, helping the body to heal itself.

There is evidence that chiropractic treatment is an effective treatment for neuromusculoskeletal disorders.

When things go wrong outside the spine

Tendinitis, earlier discussed.

The most common cause of tendinitis is overuse and repetitive motion from recreational, athletic, or occupational activities. Risk factors for tendonitis include repetitive movement, trauma, thermal injury to the tendon, use of certain antibiotics (such as levofloxacin and ciprofloxacin), and smoking. Tendinitis can also occur in people with diseases such as rheumatoid arthritis, obesity, and diabetes

Carpal tunnel,

Carpal tunnel syndrome (CTS) is a relatively common, chronic and disabling condition. This syndrome is typically characterized by nocturnal hand discomfort, finger paraesthesia in the median nerve distribution and thenar muscle atrophy.

This condition is most frequently caused by compression of the medial nerve in the carpal tunnel. This disorder occurs most often between the ages of 30 and 60 and is 2 to 5 times more common in women than men. The dominant hand is affected frequently; however, 32% to 50% of cases occur bilaterally.

Anatomically, the carpal tunnel is formed by all the carpals of the wrist, which is deepened by the tubercles of the scaphoid and trapezium on the radial side and by the pisiform and hook of the hamate on the ulnar side. This concavity is converted into a tunnel by the tough flexor retinaculum, which stretches between the tubercle of scaphoid and the ulnar styloid. The eight

45

flexors of the fingers, the long flexor of the thumb and the median nerve all share the space in the tunnel.

There are three main theories regarding the etiology of CTS:

1. The local entrapment of the median nerve within the carpal tunnel, can be classified into three groups:

   a. The decrease in the size of the carpal tunnel due to bony or soft tissue changes such as misalignment of the carpal bones, fractures, dislocation, or hypertrophic osteophytes or fibrous scarring.

   b. An increase in the volume of the normal content of the carpal tunnel. This can be due to occupational hypertrophy of the muscles and tendons in the carpal tunnel which is not uncommon in dentists, tennis and golf players, typists, factory workers, and persons confined to wheelchairs. Synovial proliferation due to arthritis, tenosynovitis, edema due to congestive heart failure, and amyloid in patients on dialysis are other less common causes for an increase in the content of the carpal tunnel.

   c. Space-occupying lesions such as lipoma and ganglion cysts will also cause entrapment of the median nerve within the carpal tunnel.

2. Systemic diseases also will cause neuritis affecting the median nerve, most commonly patients with diabetes; seven percent of patients with CTS have diabetes.

3. The third cause for CTS has been labeled as idiopathic, in fact 50% of patients with CTS have an unknown etiology. CTS has also been found in association with menopause and late trimester pregnancy.

The diagnosis of CTS until recently has been mainly empirical. Present diagnostic parameters include clinical history, clinical signs, and nerve conduction studies which can be equivocal. Imaging modalities prior to magnetic resonance imaging (MRI) have been in most circumstances non-contributory, with exception of osseous lesions, such as fractures and osteophytes. Likewise, the choice of conservative or surgical treatment is largely empirical. The reason for the success or failure of conservative treatment is poorly understood, possibly because the exact cause for the symptoms is generally not established prior to treatment.

Symptoms

1. Hyperesthesia or paresthesia in the median nerve distribution (tingling, pain, and numbness). This is never in the fifth finger on close questioning. Usually worse during rest after work.

2. Weakness of the thumb with grasping or pinching.

3. Symptoms occasionally improve with shaking or rubbing the hands.

Characteristics of the Syndrome

1. More common in women.

2. More common in the working (30-50) age group.

3. Much more common in the right, or dominant hand.

4. Both hands involved one-half of the time.

5. Symptoms often after work, at night.

6. Often described as poor circulation.

7. Often described as involving the whole hand

8. Pain often referred to the forearm or arm.

Physical Findings

1. Hypersthesia of the median nerve distribution. Use sterile or alcohol clean needle for examination or light touch.
2. Atrophy of thenar muscles (late).
3. Weakness of five-finger pinch with thumb.
4. Tinel's sign - paresthesia with digital percussion (tapping) directly on the median nerve.
5. Phalen's sign - paresthesia produced by two minutes of maximal flexion of the wrist joint.
6. Increased pain or paresthesia with arm blood pressure cuff over systolic blood pressure one to two minutes.
7. EMG usually reveals increased conduction delay (latency).
8. Primarily, CTS is a clinical diagnosis. The EMG is occasionally normal with CTS and may be abnormal in employees without symptoms.

Treatment:

Treatment of carpal tunnel syndrome can vary based on the severity of the case and the physician you are choosing. Most cases will respond to conservative treatment including cold laser, EMS, stretching and ice. Special vitamins with a certain part off the B complex and also Inositol can greatly relieve the pain and help the nerves to heal. More advance cases may require surgery in which the band overlying the tunnel is cut, allowing more room for the nerves.

Frozen shoulder

Frozen shoulder, medically referred to as **adhesive capsulitis**, is a disorder in which the shoulder capsule, the connective tissue surrounding the glenohumeral joint of the shoulder, becomes inflamed and stiff, greatly restricting motion and causing chronic pain.

Adhesive capsulitis is a painful and disabling condition that often causes great frustration for patients and caregivers due to slow recovery. Movement of the shoulder is severely restricted. Pain is usually constant, worse at night, when the weather is colder, and along with the restricted movement can make even small tasks impossible. Certain movements can cause sudden onset of tremendous pain and cramping that can last several minutes.

This condition, for which an exact cause is unknown, can last from five months to three years or more and is thought in some cases to be caused by injury or trauma to the area. It is believed that it may have an autoimmune component, with the body attacking healthy tissue in the capsule. There is also a lack of fluid in the joint, further restricting movement.

In addition to difficulty with everyday tasks, people who suffer from adhesive capsulitis usually experience problems sleeping for extended periods due to pain that is worse at night and restricted movement/positions. The condition also can lead to depression, pain, and problems in the neck and back. There are a number of risk factors for frozen shoulder, including diabetes, stroke, accidents, lung disease, connective tissue disorders, and heart disease. The condition very rarely appears in people under 40.

What causes frozen shoulder?

Most often, frozen shoulder occurs with no associated injury or discernible cause. There are patients who develop a frozen shoulder after a traumatic injury to the shoulder, but this is not the usual cause. Some risk factors for developing a frozen shoulder include:

- **Age & Gender**
  Frozen shoulder most commonly affects patients between the ages of 40 to 60 years old, and it is twice as common in women than in men.

- **Endocrine Disorders**
  Patients with diabetes are at particular risk for developing a frozen shoulder. Other endocrine abnormalities, such as thyroid problems, can also lead to this condition.

- **Shoulder Trauma or Surgery**
  Patients who sustain a shoulder injury, or undergo surgery on the shoulder can develop a frozen shoulder joint. When injury or surgery is followed by prolonged joint immobilization, the risk of developing a frozen shoulder is highest.

- **Other Systemic Conditions**
  Several systemic conditions such as heart disease and Parkinson's disease have also been associated with an increased risk for developing a frozen shoulder.

No one really understands why some people develop a frozen shoulder. For some reason, the shoulder joint becomes stiff and scarred. The shoulder joint is a ball and socket joint. The ball is the top of the arm bone (the humeral head), and the socket is part of the shoulder blade (the glenoid). Surrounding this ball-and-socket joint is a capsule of tissue that envelops the joint.

Normally, the shoulder joint allows more motion than any other joint in the body. When a patient develops a frozen shoulder, the capsule that surrounds the shoulder joint becomes contracted. The patient's body will form form bands of scar tissue called adhesions. The contraction of the capsule and the formation of the adhesions cause the frozen shoulder to become stiff and cause movement to become painful.

This condition has been described in three phases, so the symptoms will differ depending on the phase of the condition.

The Painful Phase

- Gradual onset of aching shoulder
- Developing widespread pain, often worst at night and when lying on the affected side
- This phase can last anywhere between 2-9 months

The Stiffening Phase

- Stiffness starts to become a problem
- Pain level usually does not alter
- Difficulty with normal daily tasks such as dressing, preparing food, carrying bags, working
- Muscle wastage may be evident due to lack of use
- This stage can last between 4-12 months

The Thawing Phase

- Gradual improvement in range of movement
- Gradual decrease in pain, although it may re-appear as stiffness eases
- This stage can last between 5-12 months

Treatments: Frozen shoulders can be difficult to treat and almost always take a long time to heal. Conservative treatment with laser, stretching and manipulation can greatly improve mobility. These treatments can be painful during the acute phase.

If conservative treatment is not helpful, or too painful to do in the practitioner's office, which is common, then manipulation under anesthesia may be beneficial. Manipulation under anesthesia will allow the patient to relax and not feel the pain of the range of motion exercises and movements that will allow the shoulder to regain it motion in only twenty minutes, versus three months of in-office treatments. See later in the book on MUA for more information.

Fibromyalgia

Fibromyalgia is a mysterious condition that causes pain and stiffness in the soft tissues (muscles, tendons, ligaments) and fatigue, along with many other symptoms The cause is unknown.

Fibromyalgia does not involve inflammation or muscle damage. It cannot be diagnosed with a blood test or x-ray. (Blood tests may be taken to rule out other conditions) Diagnosis is based upon the symptoms.

Many of the symptoms of fibromyalgia are seen in other disorders such as clinical depression, chronic fatigue syndrome, low thyroid function, etc. The most distinctive symptom of fibromyalgia is the presence of tender points, which are specific spots on the body that are painful when pressure is applied.

What are the Symptoms

Widespread musculoskeletal pain (that has been present for at least three months) and fatigue are the main symptoms of fibromyalgia. There are 18 specific tender points associated with fibromyalgia (areas of the body that are painful when pressed). There must be pain in at least 11 out of 18 of these points to be diagnosed with this disease. (Some doctors believe these guidelines are too rigid – what if the person has only 9 or 10 tender points but many other symptoms) A person with fibromyalgia is usually not aware of these tender points until a physician presses on them.

Sleep disorders are common (affecting 90% of patients). Even if a sufferer gets enough hours of sleep, the time spent in deep sleep – the restorative stage – is often inadequate. Many fibromyalgia sufferers also suffer from depression and/or anxiety. It is not known if this is due to the stress of chronic pain and fatigue, or if there is an actual link between these disorders. There may be headaches, and impaired memory, irritable bowel, along with many other symptoms.

The symptoms and their intensity vary from person to person. Even in the same person, symptoms may fluctuate.

The pain may range from aching to burning or gnawing pain. The intensity and location of the pain may from vary day-to-day. The neck, shoulders, lower back, and upper chest are commonly affected. Pain and stiffness are often the worst in the morning. Certain activities, overexertion, stress, damp weather, etc. may trigger increases in pain. However, the pain often fluctuates for no apparent reason.

The cause of fibromyalgia is currently unknown. However, several hypotheses have been developed. The most current theory involves the "central sensitization." This theory proposes that fibromyalgia patients have a lower threshold for pain because of an increased sensitivity or sensitization in the brain to pain signals.

Genetic predisposition

There is evidence that genetic factors may play a role in the development of fibromyalgia. For example, there is a high aggregation of fibromyalgia in families. The mode of inheritance is currently unknown, but it is most probably polygenic. Research has demonstrated that fibromyalgia is associated with polymorphisms of genes in the serotoninergic, dopaminergic and catecholaminergic systems. However, these polymorphisms are not specific for fibromyalgia and are associated with a variety of allied disorders (e.g. chronic fatigue syndrome, irritable bowel syndrome) and with depression.

Treatments: Thousands of treatments options are available for patients with fibromyalgia, including medications, nutrition, chiropractic, massage, and many others. Due to the fact that each case is so different per patient makes it difficult to make any broad recommendations.

Headaches

There are two ways to categorize headaches:

Primary Headache:

Include **tension–type, migraine, cervicogenic, and cluster headaches** and are not caused by other underlying medical conditions. More than 90% of headaches are primary.

Secondary Headache:

Result from other medical conditions, such as infection or increased pressure in the skull due to a tumor. These account for fewer than 10% of all headaches.

Descriptions of the Primary Headache Types:

1. Tension–type Headaches Tension type headaches are the most common, affecting upwards of 75% of all headache sufferers. As many as 90% of adults have had tension–type headaches.

Tension–type headaches usually involve a steady ache, rather than a throbbing one, are described as a feeling of pressure or tightening, may last minutes to days, affect both sides of the head, and do not worsen with routine physical activity. It may also be accompanied by photophobia or phonophobia (hypersensitivity to light and noise, respectively.). Nausea is usually absent. Some people get tension–type (and migraine) headaches in response to stressful events. Tension–type headaches may also be chronic, occurring frequently or daily. Psychological factors have been overemphasized as causes of headaches.

Tension headaches can be divided into three categories, according to how often they occur.

Infrequent episodic — headaches occur less than once per month

Frequent episodic — headaches occur 1-14 times per month

Chronic — headaches are present 15 days or more in a month

Rebound Headache: Rebound headache may occur among people with tension–type headaches, as well as in those with migraines. It appears to be the result of taking prescription or nonprescription pain relievers daily or almost every day, contrary to directions on the package label. If prescription or nonprescription pain relievers are overused, headache may "rebound" as the last dose wears off, leading one to take more and more pills. This is a great reason to call your chiropractor. Break that cycle!

Cervicogenic Headaches: Cervicogenic headache originates from disorders of the neck and is recognized as a referred pain in the head. Primary sensory afferents from the cervical nerve roots C_1–C_3 converge with afferents from the occiput and trigeminal afferents on the same second order neuron in the upper cervical spine. Consequently, the anatomical structures innervated by the cervical roots C_1–C_3 are potential sources of cervicogenic headache.

Cervical headache is often precipitated by neck movement and/or sustained awkward head positioning (such as painting the ceiling, or washing the floor) and can reproduced with pressure over the upper cervical or occipital region on the symptomatic side. It is often accompanied by restricted cervical range of motion, ipsilateral neck, shoulder, or arm pain of a rather vague non-radicular nature or, occasionally, arm pain of a radicular nature.

Migraine Headaches: Migraine headaches are less common than tension–type headaches. Nevertheless, migraines afflict 25 to 30 million people in the United States. As many as 6% of all men, and up to 18% of all women experience a migraine headache at some time.

Among the most distinguishing features is the potential disability accompanying the headache pain of a migraine: migraines may last 4-72 hours, are typically unilateral (60% of reported cases), throbbing, of moderate to severe intensity, and are aggravated by routine physical activity.

Nausea, with or without vomiting, and/or sensitivity to light and sound often accompany migraines. An "aura" may occur before head pain begins—involving a disturbance in vision, and/or an experience of brightly colored or blinking lights in a pattern that moves across the field of vision. About one in five migraine sufferers experiences an aura.

Usually, migraine attacks are occasional, or sometimes as often as once or twice a week, but rarely occur daily.

1. Cluster Headaches Cluster headaches are relatively rare, affecting about 1% of the population. They are distinct from migraine and tension–type headaches. Most cluster headache sufferers are male – about 85%

Cluster headaches come in groups or clusters lasting weeks or month. The pain is extremely severe but the attack is brief, lasting no more than an hour or two. The pain centers around one eye; this eye may be inflamed and watery. There may also be nasal congestion on the affected side of the face.

These "alarm clock" headaches may strike in the middle of the night, and often occur at about the same time each day during the course of a cluster. A history of heavy smoking and drinking is common, and alcohol often triggers attacks.

A study done by Duke University found that chiropractic care relieved more headaches than medications, physical therapy, or acupuncture. A strict tension-type headache is easily relieved with chiropractic care; however, different types of headaches may need further intervention such as nutrition and sometimes even medications. It is important to have your headaches evaluated, because certain headaches can indicate a more serious condition.

Knee problems,

Knee pain is caused by trauma, misalignment, and degeneration as well as by conditions like arthritis. The most common knee disorder is generally known as patellofemoral syndrome. The majority of minor cases of knee pain can be treated at home with rest and ice but more serious injuries do require surgical care.

One form of patellofemoral syndrome involves a tissue-related problem that creates pressure and irritation in the knee between the patella and the trochlea (patellar compression syndrome), which causes pain. The second major class of knee disorder involves a tear, slippage, or dislocation that impairs the structural ability of the knee to balance the leg (patellofemoral instability syndrome). Patellofemoral instability syndrome may cause either pain, a sense of poor balance, or both.

Age also contributes to disorders of the knee. Particularly in older people, knee pain frequently arises due to osteoarthritis. In addition, weakening of tissues around the knee may contribute to the problem. Patellofemoral instability may relate to hip abnormalities or to tightness of surrounding ligaments.

Cartilage lesions can be caused by:

- Accidents (fractures)
- Injuries
- The removal of a meniscus
- Anterior cruciate ligament injury
- Posterior cruciate ligament injury
- Considerable strain on the knee.

Any kind of work during which the knees undergo heavy stress may also be detrimental to cartilage. This is especially the case in professions in which people frequently have to walk, lift, or squat. Other causes of pain may be excessive on, and wear of, the knees, in combination with such things as muscle weakness and overweight.

Common complaints:

- A painful, blocked, locked or swollen knee.
- Sufferers sometimes feel as if their knees are about to give way, or may feel uncertain about their movement.

The pain felt by people with cartilage injury does not come from the cartilage itself, but from the irritated tissue surrounding the cartilage, or from pieces of cartilage that have come loose. If cartilage injury goes untreated, the layer of cartilage will continue to gradually wear away, causing arthrosis and gradual immobility.

Ankle

Ankle tendonitis is an inflammatory condition that often affects active and flat-footed individuals. Ankle tendonitis affects the posterior tibialis tendon. The posterior tibialis tendon runs underneath the "bony knob" in your ankle (see diagram below). The role of this tendon is to raise the arch of the foot. Ankle tendonitis should not be confused with Achilles tendonitis as they affect different tendons.

Ankle Tendonitis Causes

Ankle tendonitis is caused by excess stress being placed on the posterior tibialis tendon. Those most at risk of developing the condition are people involved in sports that involve a lot of stopping, starting and sharp movements and those that are not properly conditioned to physical exercise. Sports like basketball, squash, baseball, tennis and football put a lot of strain on the ankles.

Individuals who are just beginning a new exercise program often develop ankle tendonitis. The tendons around the ankle are not conditioned for exercise and inflammation can easily occur. For steps you should take to prevent ankle tendonitis see the treatment section below.

In some very rare cases ankle tendonitis can develop from genetic abnormalities. The condition may also develop with age. As the human body ages the tendons lose their elasticity and become tight. This makes them more prone to injury and tendonitis.

Ankle Tendonitis Symptoms

As with all types of tendonitis, ankle tendonitis symptoms will start off very mild during or after an activity but may develop if left untreated. The main symptoms include:

1. Pain and tenderness in the tendon with close proximity to the ankle

2. The pain is often worse during or after activity or exercise.

3. Pain in the area in the mornings and at night (advanced tendonitis)

4. Swelling, tenderness, redness and hot feeling around the area where the tendon meets the ankle

5. Stiffness during and after activity. When ankle tendonitis develops further, this stiffness may be felt throughout the entire day

6. Inability to bend your ankle and tilt your foot inwards without pain

You may feel one or all of these symptoms if you have ankle tendonitis. In most cases, the pain will develop around activity and will subside a short time afterwards. This does not mean the tendonitis is cured. This is a sign that it is developing and steps should be taken to prevent tendonitis from developing further.

Tennis elbow

What is Tennis Elbow?

Tennis elbow (epicondylitis) was first recognized by doctors more than 100 years ago and it is estimated that up to half of all tennis players will suffer from the condition at some point. Tennis elbow is the inflammation of the tendons in the elbow area and is caused by overuse and injury. Tennis elbow almost always affects the tendons out the outside of the elbow.

Treatments

Chiropractic Manipulation

This is the largest non-drug healing profession in the world.

Chiropractors are trained in a variety of adjustment techniques. Some are done by hand; some require the use of specialized instruments. Since each patient is different, your chiropractor will choose the best technique for your condition.

Some common adjustment techniques used by chiropractors include the following:

- **Motion Palpation** - this hand-on procedure is done to determine if your vertebrae are moving freely in their normal planes of motion.

- **Lumbar Roll** -the chiropractor positions the patient on his or her side, then applies a quick and precise thrust to the misaligned vertebra, returning it to its proper position.

- **Release Work** - the chiropractor applies gentle pressure using his or her fingertips to separate the vertebrae.

- **Table adjustments** - The patient lies on a special table with a "drop piece". The chiropractor applies a quick thrust at the same time the table drops. The dropping of the table allows for a lighter adjustment without the twisting positions that can accompany the manual adjustment.

- **Instrument adjustments** - often the gentlest methods of adjusting the spine. The patient lies on the table face down while the chiropractor uses a string-loaded activator instrument to perform the adjustment. This technique is often used to perform adjustments on animals as well.

Chiropractic Treatment For Back Pain Relief

There is evidence that chiropractic relieves many types of back pain, lower back pain in particular, and helps restore normal range of motion. Spinal manipulations may take stress off surrounding tissues - muscles, tendons, and ligaments - to relieve back pain and restore normal functioning. Some chiropractors follow scientific guidelines and only do manipulations for people with neuromusculoskeletal problems. These chiropractors often work with doctors in treating back pain.

What does a chiropractor do to relieve back pain?

Chiropractors correct subluxation by manipulation of the vertebrae (and sometimes other areas of the body). Chiropractors call this an adjustment. Spinal adjustments are usually done manually, the chiropractor using his or her hands to apply pressure to the spine to coax the vertebrae into proper alignment. Some use high velocity thrusts. Chiropractors usually massage and stretch muscles before doing an adjustment. Some apply spinal traction. This allows the vertebrae to be more easily manipulated.

Some chiropractors offer physical therapy as well as spinal manipulation. A chiropractor may also give advice on ergonomics, exercise, and proper body mechanics to prevent back pain. Chiropractors often give their patients stretching and strengthening exercises to do, as lengthening and strength-ening various muscle groups help keep the spine in proper alignment.

Chiropractic Treatment and Massage Therapy go hand in hand for back pain relief

Chiropractors often work with massage therapists in treating back pain. Tight, tense muscles can pull the vertebrae out of alignment. Once the chiropractor has made an adjustment to the spine, stretching the muscles can help keep the adjustment in place. It is also difficult for the chiropractor to perform an adjustment on a person who has tense back muscles. A multi-treatment approach to relieving back pain has often has the best success rate.

What is that popping sign when I get adjusted?

*Pockets of gas escaping from the spinal joints cause the pop-ping noise heard during a spinal adjustment and is not evidence that the vertebrae were out of alignment.

Chiropractic treatment, alone or in conjunction with other therapies, has been shown to effectively relieve back pain and help restore normal range of motion. As with any treatment, results vary from person to person.

Ultrasound

Therapeutic ultrasound is a form of deep heat therapy created by sound waves. When applied to soft tissues and joints, the sound waves are a form of micro-massage that help reduce swelling, in-crease blood flow, and decrease pain, stiffness, and spasms. Ultrasound is useful for any conditions with inflammation, including tennis elbow, tendonitis, or inflamaiton in the spine.

Electric Muscle stimulation

TENS (transcutaneous electrical nerve stimulation) devices can perform a useful function by providing an alternate tingling sensation to the pain that blocks the pain signal to the brain. Point stimulation, a newer form of electrical stimulation, may work similarly to acupuncture in providing pain relief. All forms of electrical stimulation can be placed at trigger points or at the site of pain.

Other forms of muscle stimulation are also used in the office setting. TENS machines are primarily for at home use, while in office stronger machines are available including interferntial, galvanic, and low volt. Different electricic properties are used to achieve different results. These therapies are mostly good for muscle relaxation, spasm control, and in any situation where there is muscular tension. These therapies work particularly well for sprain strain types of injuries.

Hot/cold Therapy

Heat therapy is useful for back spasms or other conditions. A meta-analysis of studies by the Cochrane Collaboration concluded that heat therapy can reduce symptoms of acute and sub-acute low-back pain. Some patients find that moist heat works best (e.g. a hot bath or whirlpool) or continuous low-level heat (e.g. a heat wrap that stays warm for 4 to 6 hours).

Heat can be applied in several different ways. Hot towels or heating pads applied directly to the pain site or hot baths can increase blood flow and soothe tensed and spasming muscles. Moist heat generally penetrates more deeply; several microwavable hot packs are now available, allowing for quicker application and convenience. Diathermy stimulates deep muscle heat by means of an electric current applied lightly to the surface of the skin. Ultrasound also elevates tissue temperature by penetrating deeply into the muscle with high-frequency sound waves. Popular heat-generating devices are two hands.

Ice and heat have long been used to treat many painful conditions. Ice therapy is often used to reduce swelling and help control pain immediately after an injury. Heat therapy is used to relax the muscles, increase circulation, and can provide relief to patients with chronic pain. Depending on the patient's condition, a combination of ice and heat can be used.

Traction

Spinal Traction is constant or intermittent pulling force applied to the spine to gradually stretch the spine. Traction stretches muscles and ligaments and increases the space between the vertebrae.

Many chiropractors and physical therapists use traction in conjunction with other treatments to relieve chronic lower back pain, especially sciatica.

Traction can relieve pressure on compressed nerves, help muscles relax, and reduce muscle spasms. Traction increases the space between vertebrae - reducing pressure on intervertebral discs and nerve root. The vertebral separation is temporary, but may last long enough to allow some patients to exercise without aggravating sciatica.

The therapist must decide the optimum amount of force to use and the length of time the force is sustained. Enough force must be used to cause vertebral separation. Though relatively safe, excessive force could increase pain or injury. Force is increased slowly to avoid overstretching or triggering muscle spasms. Traction should not cause pain although mild soreness is often felt the next day.

There are different techniques used in lumbar traction, both mechanical and manual. Inversion therapy is a form of traction that uses a person's own body weight and gravity to stretch the spine. Inversion therapy can be performed at home but should not be done without approval from a physician.

Spinal Decompression Therapy

Spinal Decompression therapy is not for every patient. Only certain patients with certain diagnosis can be treated using spinal decompression. Spinal decompression is best used to treat lumbar stenosis, or the narrowing of the spinal column due to age and degeneration, bulging discs, herniated discs and other treatments that cannot be treated using traditional conservative care.

Spinal Decompression involves tractioning a patients spine, while stabilizing them, with specific computer controlled pulls and rests, which allow the spine to open and close. This opening and closing motion allows the vertebrae to open up slowly, over time, to allow for more room for the nerves without surgery. It also is used to rehydrate the discs of the spine, and may allow disc bulges and herniations to move slightly back to place. MRI studies have confirmed that discs can rehydrate and can be decreased using this advanced treatment. There are many imposter machines that do not do real decompression and only do traction. Decompression is a specialized treatment, using a very sophisticated computer controlled device to precisely decompress a specific spinal level. You should seek a physician who is uniquely trained in this device and only if they have the best equipment available. Again, decompression is a treatment not meant for everyone, but can greatly benefit and possible save the right patient from surgery.

Cervical Traction

Cervical spinal traction is accepted as effective treatment for short-term relief of neck pain. It can relieve muscle spasm and nerve root compression by stretching soft tissues and increasing the spaces between cervical vertebrae.

Home cervical traction should not be done without approval from a physician, and preferably under the supervision of a physical therapist or other medical professional. Inexpensive over-the-door home cervical traction devices, which uses a pulley system with attached weights, provides up to 20 pounds of traction. There are pneumatic traction devices that can be used at home that employ up to 50 pounds of force. These devices generally require a prescription and complete instruction on use by a chiropractic physician.

Stretching

Therapeutic Stretches

Following an injury, therapeutic stretching is an important way to prevent scar tissue from forming. Even after the injury has healed, maintaining a regular stretching program helps keep tissues flexible, increases mobility, and protects you from new injuries. As with exercise, your chiropractor will instruct you on proper stretching techniques and will supervise you until you are comfortable enough to do them on your own.

Cold Laser Therapy

A variety of names have been used to describe the same type of low-level laser: biostimulation, low energy, low reactive, low intensity, soft and/or cold laser. In current practice, Low Level Laser Therapy uses low output levels (15100 mW), short treatment times (10-240 seconds), and low energy levels (1-4 J/cm2).[1]

The mechanism and effectiveness of LLLT has been compared with ultrasound therapy, and should be considered as an extension to the accepted physiotherapy modalities that currently utilize parts of the electromagnetic spectrum, such as shortwaves, microwaves, infrared, and ultraviolet therapy.

Lasers produce non-ionizing, electromagnetic radiation that is extremely monochromatic, polarized and coherent. Laser light has been reported to penetrate human tissue in the ranges of .8-15mm, but the majority of the light will be absorbed within the first 4mm. Although this may seem superficial, it should be noted that chemical processes may be initiated and mediate physiological effects at a deeper level.

Low-level laser therapy is the application of visible red or near-infrared light emitted from a low power laser for therapeutic purposes.

Low-level laser therapy is used to help heal wounds and to treat many of types of musculoskeletal injuries and disorders including back pain caused by lower back strain, herniated discs, fibromyalgia, etc.

Low-level lasers operate at **very low** levels of power. Unlike high-power lasers, low-level lasers do not heat or damage human tissue.

The laser device is held against the skin over the area being treated. Low-level lasers emit wavelengths of light in the visible red to near-infrared red range, which penetrate deeply into the tissues.

The light energy is absorbed and converted to biochemical energy, which stimulates the cells. Low-level laser therapy is believed to speed healing and reduce pain and inflammation. There are no known side effects to low-level laser therapy.

Low-level laser therapy is used to treat both acute and chronic pain. The benefits of low-level laser therapy appear to be cumulative - it may take several treatments for the results to become evident.

Total number of treatments needed depends upon the condition being treated, the severity of the condition, and each patient's individual response.

How does laser light differ from "natural" light?

'Natural' light (including sunlight, common light bulbs, LEDs) emits incoherent light in almost all directions over a wide spectrum of wavelengths.

Laser light is coherent (highs and low points of waves are lined up). The light waves from a laser are parallel (travel in the almost the same direction) to produce a small, concentrated beam of light. Laser light is monochromatic, meaning a laser emits light at one or more specific wavelengths rather than a wide range of wavelengths.

Different wavelengths of light have different biological effects. Wavelengths of light in the **visible red to near-infrared red range** penetrate deeply into the tissues. The light energy is absorbed and converted to biochemical energy.

Clinical Studies

A number of papers have shown a reduction of pain with laser treatments directed over acupuncture points. Altered skin resistance with a reduction of pain were also noted in subjects who receive LLLT over muscular trigger points.

A group of subjects with chronic tendinopathies that had been previously treated unsuccessfully with physical therapy, NSAIDS, local injections, and/or surgery, had an 87 percent success rate in pain reduction following the application of LLLT.

In a study involving over 4,000 subjects who had suffered from conditions such as degenerative arthritis, muscle pain, tendinitis, and tension myalgia, more than 80 percent of the subjects found a marked lessening of their symptoms following irradiation with an IR laser.

In a study involving a total of 69 subjects and 302 total laser treatment sessions, more that 80 percent of the subjects with chronic radiculopathies and over 90 percent of the subjects with chronic neuropathies experienced a greater than 50 percent total relief of pain following LLLT. In a similar study involving 60 total patients and 111 total laser treatments, it was shown that LLLT produced an immediate reduction of pain in 79 percent of the subjects.

In a study involving over 100 subjects and over 500 laser treatments, it was observed that acute soft tissue pain syndromes showed a dramatic response following the initial laser treatment with a marked reduction in tissue swelling, bruising and good pain relief. Subsequent treatments (2-3) produced further improvement. It was also noted that chronic pain syndromes were slower to respond to LLLT (average of eight treatments), although 75 percent of the subjects noted significant pain relief.

A two-stage survey of 116 chartered physiotherapists in Northern Ireland, who utilize LLLT as part of their clinical practice, ranked LLLT effective for the treatment of myofascial and postoperative pain syndromes; rheumatoid arthritis; muscle tears; hematomas; tendinitis; shingles; herpes simplex; scarring; burn and would healing. In this same survey, LLLT was ranked first, on the basis of relative effectiveness, when compared with four other modalities (interferential therapy, shortwave diathermy, ultrasound, and pulsed electromagnetic therapy), for use in pain relief and wound healing.

Chiropractic Wellness

Chiropractic treatment methods are used for pain relief and to help with acute problems, however, many people have found a chiropractic lifestyle can help in many other ways. Thousands of patients see a chiropractor on a regular basis, once a week, once a month, or as needed, in order to enjoy a healthy lifestyle, perform and feel their best. Patients who go to chiropractic regularly report feeling more energy, having less problems, less allergies, less stress, and a better quality of life. Adjusting the spine on a regular basis helps keep the joints moving properly, helps lubricate the spine, and helps the nerves remain interference free. I often tell my patients that if they only had one car for the rest of their life, how good of care would they take? I bet you would get regular oil changes, check the fluids and do all the maintenance the car needed. I bet you would drive it for ten years without changing the oil or filling the gas tank would you? Well, guess what, this is the only body you have, so you better take care of it! Millions of people have found that regular chiropractic visits help to live their life to the fullest!

Nutrition 101

While most of us know that good nutrition is essential in helping us feel our best and reach our optimal health; finding time to eat a balanced diet on a daily basis seems a formidable task in this fast-paced, affluent society. Yet, though your life may be hectic, there are still many good tasting, healthy choices which can help you lose weight and improve your health. This information is designed to be a practical guide in finding those choices whether you are at home, at work, on the road, or at a friend's home. The good news is that by taking charge of your diet, you can improve your health while reducing your risk of "lifestyle" diseases such as heart disease or cancer.

A good place to start is defining what constitutes a "healthy" diet. The "Four Food Group" Plan of yesteryear implied that foods in the Meat, Dairy, Breads and Vegetable Fruit group were equal in their contribution to a healthy diet. Today, researchers show that diets rich in complex carbohydrates and low in saturated fats may reduce our risk of chronic disease. Health professionals designed the "Food Pyramid" guide to translate these recommendations into a food plan for daily living.

Complex Carbohydrates

Complex carbohydrates are present in whole grain breads, cereals, starches and fruits and vegetables. These foods are not only rich in B vitamins and trace minerals, but they also contribute dietary fiber which has been shown to reduce risk for developing certain cancers, lowering cholesterol levels and helping in weight control.

Six to twelve servings of breads, cereals and starches may sound like a lot of food, but when you consider one cup of rice is three servings of cereal, you can see that meeting these guidelines isn't that difficult.

Fruits and Vegetables

Likewise for fruits and vegetables. Most people gag at the thought of eating four to seven servings per day until they discover one medium piece of fruit is two servings. Your typical salad is at least three servings; and let's not forget that lettuce and tomato in your deli sandwich, that counts as one also.

Proteins

Proteins are found in the dairy and meat group.

Foods in the *dairy group* not only provide protein, but they also contribute calcium, Vitamin D and other essential nutrients required for synthesizing healthy bones and teeth. They can be a significant source of saturated fat, so chose two to three servings of the low-fat (1% fat or less) milks, yogurts and/or cheeses.

The *meat group* includes chicken, fish, nuts and beans or legumes. A deck of cards roughly approximates a three ounce serving and you need at least two servings a day. These foods provide zinc, magnesium and iron which, along with protein, are used by the body in creating hemoglobin and lean body tissue. These foods can also contribute to an elevated intake of saturated fat, so chose lean cuts of meat like flank or round steak, pork tenderloin, ham and leg of lamb. Skip the skin on chicken or turkey and you will miss much of the fat and cho-

lesterol. Better yet, skip animal protein altogether and try min-
estrone or split pea soup, chili or bean burritos.

Fats and Sugar

Fats, sugars and alcohol have the least amount of surface area
on the pyramid for a reason. They contribute little more than
calories to the diet and your body will squeeze them into a fat
cell. Worse yet, your body will create another fat cell to harbor
them until they are burned.

Many health organizations, like the American Heart Association and the American Cancer Society, agree that limiting your
fat intake to less than 30% of calories goes a long way to protect you from life threatening diseases. A gram of fat has nine
calories, and that isn't much fat. As there is some fat in dairy
products and meat, chicken and fish; you are better off to avoid
adding fat to your food. Luckily, there are many good tasting
low-fat or nonfat salad and sandwich spreads which make the
task of avoiding added fat a lot easier.

Yes, certain fats are essential to good nutrition (like linoleic
acid), but these are found in ample amounts in whole grain
breads, cereals and vegetables. Corn, for example, is where
Mother Nature originally put corn oil. Why not skip the marga-
rine and just eat corn?

Summary

IN SHORT, GOOD NUTRITION means eating a wide variety of foods from each of the five food groups. The Food Pyramid shows us that by eating more complex carbohydrates and less total fat and saturated fat, we can become empowered by the good life and not fall victim to it. One of the best ways to track your diet is by use of a diet diary, allowing your self to track what you eat everyday, or better yet, go over the information with your chiropractor!

Diet and Nutritional Counseling

Studies have shown that poor diet and nutritional imbalances contribute to a number of serious illnesses, such as heart disease, stroke, diabetes, and cancer. Chiropractors are specifically trained in diet and nutritional counseling. Your chiropractor can design a nutritional program specific to your needs that can help you maintain good health and minimize the risk of developing these serious health conditions.

Lifestyle Modification Counseling

Good health is much more than the absence of pain or disease. The lifestyle choices you make on a daily basis can greatly affect your long-term health. We now know that years of seemingly small unhealthy lifestyle choices can, over time, turn into very large health problems. Examples of lifestyle choices and behaviors that can have negative effects on your health include:

- lack of regular exercise
- smoking
- poor diet
- excessive mental stress
- over-reliance on medication
- excessive consumption of alcohol
- poor posture
- improper lifting

Your chiropractor will talk to you about your lifestyle choices, help you sort through and identify unhealthy health habits, and give you practical strategies to deal with and manage them.

As you can see, chiropractic medicine is more than just spinal manipulations. Chiropractors use a variety of treatment modalities to help the body to heal itself and return the patient to a pain-free and healthy life.

Dr. Supervised only Symptom survey

Symptom Surveys are the easiest way to evaluate nutrient need. Patients simply respond to the presence or absence of symptoms and their severity. We may also take into account diet, acid/alkaline balance and basal body temperatures on this form; along with the patient and family histories.

PH and you

Monitoring your pH gives you a general indication of how well or how hard your body is working to survive your lifestyle. The results of your pH tests are indicators of how your body is responding to the foods you eat and to other stresses. The actual acid or alkaline level of your internal environment affects how your body functions.

pH has a profound effect on health and disease. Imbalances in pH mean that the body has become too acidic or too alkaline for long periods of time which is not very well tolerated by the body. In fact, the body has regulatory mechanisms (breathing, circulation, digestion, hormonal production, etc.) that serve the purpose of managing and balancing pH levels. If the pH deviates too far to the acid side or too far to the alkaline side, cells become poisoned by their own toxins and die.

Studies have shown that healthy people's body fluids are slightly alkaline while the same fluids of those who are sick are acidic, ranging from slightly acidic to extremely acidic. In Dr. Mark Cochran's book "The Secrets of pH Concerning Health and Disease" he states the body should remain in a slightly alkaline condition in order to avoid disease and premature aging.

Virtually all degenerative diseases including cancer, heart disease, arthritis, osteoporosis, kidney and gall stones, and tooth decay are associated with excess acidity in the body. While the body has a homeostatic mechanism that maintains a constant pH 7.4 in the blood, this mechanism works by depositing and withdrawing acid and alkaline minerals from other locations including the bones, soft tissues, body fluids and saliva. Therefore, the pH of these other tissues can fluctuate greatly. The pH of saliva offers a general window through which you can see the overall pH balance in your body.

Your salivary pH should stay in a range of 7.0–7.5 for healthy body function. The best time to test your salivary pH is approximately 1 hour before a meal and 2 hours after a meal. If your urinary pH fluctuates between 6.0–6.5 in the morning and between 6.5–7.0 in the evening, your body is functioning within a healthy range.

Saliva

Using your saliva as a diagnostic tool, you can implement individually appropriate changes to your life to reach optimal health. In general, saliva testing of the adrenal glands offers a powerful tool to evaluate gastrointestinal problems, stress-related and hormone-related diseases, and the overall wellness of the human body.

Saliva testing is an extremely effective diagnostic tool to improve one's health; it offers a view into the body's emotional, hormonal, immunological, nutritional and metabolic health. The extensive range of communications and relationships among these factors opens a uniquely accurate healing protocol. Optimal health is dependent on the balance of hormones and not just a single hormone at one certain time of day. Saliva is used to pick up the nuances that may not show in blood work- how many times have you heard "blood work normal" yet you have every sign and symptom that clearly shows you are not functioning normally.

Saliva testing is convenient, non-invasive and inexpensive, which allows for needed multiple tests over an extended period of time to design individual healing programs. Saliva tests the free hormones, which are the correct reflection of the bioactivity of the hormones available for use to the bodily tissues.

Blood work

Blood Chemistry can be a tool for the assessment of nutritional status within the body. In allopathic, or mainstream medical care it is the primary means for the diagnosis of disease. Blood work is an excellent indicator of the end-stage of disease. In other words, blood values are generally the last of the indicators used naturopathically to go awry. This is necessary within allopathic medicine due to the nature of their treatments. The end-stage must be reached prior to prescribing medications with side effects or potentially dangerous surgeries. This is why so many patients feel as though there is something wrong with their health but their medical doctor appears to be playing the "wait and see" game. Naturopathically, we use blood values, not to ascertain end-stages of disease, but to see optimal physiological balance. This is accomplished by using *optimal* reference ranges rather than population averages for the desired blood values.

Urine

An ordinary urine test can be used to formulate the exact state the body is in and help in devising a chiropractic solution. This is what a chiropractor would be looking for:

- Carbohydrates (sugar) in the urine, an indicator of your energy levels and available energy. Imbalances indicate liver and pancreatic function may not be optimum.

- pH of urine shows how effectively nutrients can be absorbed.

- pH of saliva shows this may be the cause of weight gain or inability to gain weight. Again this is an indication of liver and pancreatic function out of balance.

- The amount of cellular debris in the urine indicates how the body is disposing of cellular waste.

- Mineral salts in the urine indicate how well hydrated the body is.

- Nitrate Nitrogen (NN) shows how well protein is being broken down in the small intestine and is the key to your body's need for potassium. A high reading indicates a problem in the upper part of the body.

- Ammonium Nitrates (AN) indicate how much putrefactive waste is being absorbed primarily from the bowel.

- The total of your NN and AN show the level of urea being passed in the urine, another pointer to major stress factors and tiredness. These numbers also indicate where your major weakness is in the body. It also indicates infections, liver deficiencies, kidney problems, energy imbalances and dietary concerns.

Whole Food, Organic

Whole food supplements, on the other hand, provide nutrients as nature intended - in a whole food form. In this way you receive more of the nutrients the whole food provides, rather than incomplete isolated components of the food.

The body has an amazing capacity to heal itself, but it must have good nutrition. This means eating a healthy diet that includes fresh fruits and vegetables daily. It means eating healthy sources of grains and avoiding highly processed wheat and flour products. It means eating the right amount of protein from a good source. It means restricting the amounts of processed foods and fast-foods eaten. It means limiting the sweets and sugar in the diet. And it means taking high-quality whole food supplements.

Natural vitamin C helps the body heal conditions such as bleeding gums and varicose or spider veins. Synthetic vitamin

C (ascorbic acid) is made from corn sugar. Mega dosages can lead to collagen disease, impaired mineral metabolism and an imbalance with other vitamins, leading to formation of kidney stones and diabetes mellitus. Natural vitamin B (such as in rice bran) helps the body heal the nervous system. Synthetic vitamin B (thiamine) is made from coal tar and can lead to nerve damage.

Good Quality Supplements

It is important to only take good quality, whole food, organic supplements. These supplements will allow your body to heal itself, versus forcing bad nutrients into the body. Most of the supplements you buy at the local drug store, or mega discount store will do more harm than good. If your taking poor quality vitamins, your better off not taking any. For example, a well known brand many people take that begins with c, is known to derive some of its chemically derived nutraceuticals from crude oil. I don't think you want to put that into your body!

We carry and distribute only standard process supplements. Standard Process has been providing whole food supplements since the 1920s. They control the entire process from planting the seeds to the supplements, to bottling and selling the supplements. Most nutritional companies sell nutraceuticals, which as chemically derived mega dose formulas. One major manufacturer of these nutraceuticals actually uses left over crude oil to make many of its formulas. This is not nutrition. Standard process is only available at qualified health care professional offices with medical recommendations. This is medical grade, true nutrition and should be take only under direction and advice from a physician. More information can be found on their website at **http://www.standardprocess.com**

We cannot comment or give advice on any products we do not carry.

<u>Boswellia</u> Combination of natural herbs to decrease acute or new swelling and inflammation

<u>Congoplex</u> Supplement to boost immune system when you have a cold

<u>CardioPlus:</u> Combination of supplements to improve heart health

<u>Livton</u> oriental herb used to manage high cholesterol

<u>Ligaplex 1</u> special blend of vitamins and herbs to heal joints that have recently been injured

<u>Ligaplex 2</u> special blend of vitamins and herbs to heal joints that have been chronically injured

<u>Black Cohosh</u> natural herb that may help with hot flashes and menopause symptoms

<u>SP Cleanse</u> can be used alone or in our purification kit to detox the body

<u>Saligesic:</u> Natural Alternative to NSAIDS, such as Aleve, Tylenol, long term use

<u>Tuna Omega 3:</u> Naturally made from tuna, omega oils are good for anti inflation, heart health, and general health

<u>Calcium Lactate</u> Calcium and magnesium, good for bone health, heart health, and headaches

<u>Lact-Enz:</u> Naturally occurring digestive enzymes, pro-biotic. Help digestion, stomach problems, and overall health

Cataplex B: B vitamin complex, good for increased energy, nerve issues, carpal tunnel syndrome.

Catyln: Multi vitamin, good for everyone

OPC Synergy: Anti-oxidant formula, including reservatrol and other,

Drenamin: Adrenal Gland support, good for adrenal problems, low energy, ligament tightening

Immunoplex: Immune system support, take when your sick or feeling a cold coming on

Thyroid Complex: Good for thyroid support, particularly slow thyroid

Inositol: Specific part of the B complex that alleviates nerve pain

Standard Bar: Meal replacement and snack bar, take them on the go!

We carry and recommend many different supplements in addiction to these. Please consult the office for more information. This is not intended to diagnose or treat any condition. Please do not attempt a supplement plan without consulting with a qualified physician.

Herbs and Supplements

Herbal medicine is used by 80% of the world's population. People in the US are increasingly accepting it. In fact, it is now a 3.87 billion dollar industry in this country. It is growing at the rate of 25-50% each year. In Germany, since 1974, Commission E, a division of the German Federal Health Agency, has had the responsibility of reviewing herbal medicines including chemical analysis, traditional usage and scientific studies of toxicology, pharmacology and epidemiology.

What do you do if these conventional treatments haven't worked for your pain?

Either in your spine or extremities, what happens if diet, nutrition, chiropractic, physical therapy, and even medications haven't worked? Finally, a non-invasive procedure that could give you your life back?

Studies have shown that only 25 percent of patients who undergo spinal surgery feel better after 2 years? In fact 25 percent feel worse two years later?

This could be your answer!

Manipulation under anaesthesia

Monitored Anesthestic care, IV sedation- lets the body relax, not fight the manipulation, allows breakdown of scar tissue and adhesions. Patients who don't respond as well to chiropractic care may consider manipuiation under anesthesia.

Manipulation done under anesthesia (or twilight sedation) - this is performed by a chiropractor certified in this technique in a hospital outpatient setting when you are unresponsive to traditional adjustments.

Manipulation Under Anesthesia is exactly what it sounds like. After medical clearance, the patient is lightly anesthetized to achieve total relaxation, then, specialized stretching movements and adjustments which would normally be too painful to even consider are easily and painlessly accomplished. Manipulation

Under Joint Anesthesia involves the performance of specialized spinal intervention procedures in addition to the above.

For more and more patients who are not finding relief through conventional treatments and/or invasive procedures, MUA, combined with consistent but simple post-procedure treatment and exercise regimen, can eliminate or greatly reduce pain and restore or markedly improve range of motion. Plus, MUA procedures are cost-effective - thousands of dollars less than traditional surgery and other more invasive treatments - and usually qualify for insurance coverage.

In addition, return-to-work is much faster, allowing MUA patients to get back to work and the pleasures of living much sooner than expected.

IS MUA/MUJA NEW OR EXPERIMENTAL?

MUA is neither new nor experimental. It's actually been practiced since the late 1930's and used by osteopathic physicians and orthopedic surgeons for many years as a proven form of treatment.

During the past eight years, interest in MUA has greatly increased thanks to tremendous advances in anesthesiology.

Today, MUA is a multi-disciplinary outpatient procedure that takes place in a controlled hospital or ambulatory surgical setting, usually over the course of one to three days.

Using specialized techniques, supported by the expertise of MDs, RNs, Chiropractors and Anesthesiologists, MUA achieves maximum results for qualified patients.

Countless recent case studies and medical research continue to show that MUA is widely regarded as safe and effective and is gaining acceptance by the medical community at large.

WHO CAN BENEFIT FROM MUA/MUJA?

MUA can be a valuable procedure for people with chronic neck, back and joint problems - conditions caused by long-term disabilities, accidents, and injuries that have not been responsive to conventional treatment but MUA is not for everybody. Please contact your physician for details.

Common, general conditions that MUA could be effective in include:

Degenerative Disc Disease
Herniated Nucleus Pulposus
Chronic myofascitis
Neuromusculoskeletal conditions
Failed Back Surgery Syndrome
Fibro adhesion buildup
Myofascial Pain Syndrome
Spinal Stenosis
Osteoarthritis

Patients who have reached a plateau using conservative care/surgical care/chiropractic care/physical therapy can significantly improve their quality of life using MUA.

WHY DOES MUA/MUJA WORK?

MUA achieves results where other treatments fail because it allows your caregivers to use a sophisticated biomechanical approach for the neuromusculoskeletal system.

"Twilight" sedation allows you to be responsive, but not apprehensive. This also helps to preserve the natural protective reflexes of the body.

Specialized stretching and manipulations are completed gently, and without the patient's usual pain trained physical or psychological resistance.

Fibrotic adhesions, which limit range of motion and contribute to pain, are altered; muscles are stretched; collagen fibers are remodeled to eliminate or reduce restriction. Pain and discomfort are decreased.

The manual medicine techniques utilized during MUA require less force because of the relaxed state and are more physiologically suitable.

HOW DO I BEGIN AN MUA/MUJA TREATMENT PLAN?

Once proper patients are selected using standards of care as described by the National Academy of MUA Physicians, the typical MUA treatment plan begins with a medical screening process to clear the patient for anesthesia. Medical tests usually will include but are not limited to:

CBC
Metabolic Panel
Chest X-ray and EKG
Electrocardiogram
Pregnancy test for Female MUA/MUJA patients
Other Necessary Testing

Additional tests, such as MRI/CT and other diagnostic tests as necessary.

After receiving medical clearance, the patient is scheduled at the facility where the MUA will be performed.

WHAT'S THE MUA/MUJA PROCEDURE LIKE?

On the day of the MUA, the patient must be accompanied by a friend or family member to drive the patient home after the procedure. No patient will be allowed to drive following this procedure.

The patient then confers with the anesthesiologist, is gowned and the sedative - usually Diprivan and/or Versed, and sometimes Fentanyl - are administered to achieve the comfortable sleep that makes treatment possible.

MUA begins with specialized stretching and adjustment techniques that are used in the spine segments affected. Specialized interventional procedures are performed as necessary for MUJA.

WHAT HAPPENS AFTER THE PROCEDURE?

After the procedure is completed, the patient is repositioned and awakened, and then taken to the recovery room where he or she is carefully monitored by the O.R, nurse.

Recovery time is generally 10 to 20 minutes. After recovery, the patient receives oral fluids and a light snack. The doctor and anesthesiologist also remain in attendance until the patient is discharged.

To achieve results in most chronic cases, the MUA procedure is repeated. The doctor may adjust only the area of abnormality, plus the adjacent area, the adjacent area only or additional areas depending on the doctor's assessment of the condition.

Post-procedure care is one of the most import parts of the MUA procedure and makes it truly effective.

The therapy begins immediately after MUA procedure is completed. At this time, the patient visits the office and undergoes a combination of stretching exercises, cryo-therapy and electrical stimulation to eliminate or reduce soreness. The patient then returns home to rest.

Following the last MUA procedure, the patient should follow an intensive therapy program for seven to 10 days. This post MUA therapy should be the same stretches accomplished during the MUA procedure and necessary adjustments made in the doctor's office.

This is followed by specific rehabilitation for the next two to three weeks including stretching, flexibility and strengthening exercises plus periodic adjustments as required by the doctor.

A regimented program of post-MUA therapy will help the patient regain both pre-injury strength and help prevent future pain and disability.

Training

Manipulation under anesthesia is similar to regular chiropractic manipulation; however, the procedure requires advanced training that must be taken by any doctor who performs the procedure. Chiropractors, Osteopaths, or Medical Doctors can all perform the procedure if they have taken the certification course, passed two written exams and successfully passed a proctorship involving supervised procedures. The training is intensive and there are a few select doctors who have completed the necessary training.

Research

1. 83 % of patients with EMG verified radiculopathies reported significant improvement – Robert Mensor, M.D.

2. Patients that had back pain for a minimum of 10 years reported an 87% recovery rate after MUA –Ongly et al

3. 51 % of patients with unrelieved symptoms after conservative care had been exhausted reported good to excellent results three years post MUA –Donald Christman, MD

4. 71 % of 723 MUA patients had good results (returned to normal activity relatively symptom free) and flexibility, elasticity and range of motion can be resorted following MUA –Bradford and Siehl

5. 83% of 517 patients treated with MUA responded well. – Paul Kuo, MD Professor of Orthopedic surgery

6. 171 Patients who had constant intractable pain for several months to 18 years. All patients had failed conservative treatment. The study showed that 25% of patients had no pain following MUA, 50% were much improved, and 20% were better and could tolerate the pain. Failures were less than 5 % with little or no pain relief. –Krumhansi and Nowacek

7. 64 % of patients with a herniated disc reported good to excellent results –Merril C. Mensor, MD

8. 96.3% of patient diagnosed with myofibrositis (muscle tissue scarring and adhesions) reported good to excellent results.

Manipulation under anesthesia is not for everyone. This treatment option is only for certain types of well-qualified patients. Patient selection is very important for obtaining proper results. However, if you have had chronic pain, and you haven't seen relief. This may be the treatment option you have been looking for. For more information on MUA, visit my website, http://www.villagefamilychiro.com, or call my main office at 908-813-8200, and ask for a free MUA consult.

What the Doctor Did to Me !!!

I HAD SCIATICA PROBLEMS for about 7 years, and severe **sinus problems** for 2 years. I never saw any other doctors; I just suffered through it. Positive results became apparent after my second or third chiropractic visit. **I felt like a weight was lifted off my shoulders right after my first visit.**

DAWN E. QUIRK, Hackettswon, NJ, independent business woman

When I first came to your office I was apprehensive about if you would be able to help me, where all of my other doctors had failed. To my amazement, you were the doctor I had been waiting for to end my suffering. I have had terrible pains in my upper thighs over the past year. My primary care physician said to lose weight and I would feel better. I lost the weight and nothing happened. One of the best decisions I have ever made was walking into your office. You treated me as an individual, you were thorough, and did not force me into treatments. **You gave me back my life and pain free days**. I look forward to finishing my treatments with you, and would recommend your practice to anyone.

P.S. Your staff have been so nice and very understanding. They are great people.

MICHAEL GANZ, belvidere, student

I came into your office unable to stand upright or walk more than fifty feet without terrible pain in both my right leg and back. I faithfully came to your office three times a week and showed improvement after each visit. After six weeks of chiropractic care, I am well on the road to recovery. The sciatica pain has disappeared and my lower back is feeling stronger every day. I was disappointed that my family doctor offered nothing but pain medication, but your proactive approach obviously worked. **I want to thank you and your staff for working with me and improving my back condition**.

RICHARD YOCUM, Jefferson, new jersey, business manager

I suffered from cramps, cold symptoms and joint aches. The cramps and cold symptoms stopped after receiving chiropractic adjustments. As for the Arthritis- there is less need for medication with continued chiropractic care. **I am in good condition for a woman of 80 years**.

ELOISE MIAL, Belvidere NJ, retired

I had knee, leg, and foot pain for about three months. **After approximately 3 weeks of treatment from Dr. Fedich, I was able to do my daily walks**, more gardening, and am not bothered at night with pain.

MILSIE CARPENTER, Hackettstown, NJ, retired

Lower back pain was my problem. I could not bend down without experiencing severe pain. After two weeks of coming to your office, the pain was alleviated. **This was my first experience with chiropractic. I am convinced that it works.**

Dr. BEN ADAMS, Allamuchy, NJ psychologist

I experienced heal pain for a year, and my lower arm had begun to hurt for two months. I was unable to walk to do my normal chores or to raise my arm for normal lifting. After a month I began to feel better. After just a few months, **I am able to walk without pain and have no pain in my arm**. Dr. Fedich is very caring and that, in itself; makes you feel better.

GRACE J. CLEGG, Andover, NJ, retired

I had problems with my neck that prevented me from being able to participate in school sports. After just two weeks, I noticed results. **Dr. Fedich helped me quickly and painlessly**.

MICHAEL SOARES, Long Valley, NJ, student

I want to express my gratitude for helping my daughter, Beth, feel a lot better. She had constant lower back, shoulder, and neck pain, but was not eager to start her sessions since we all are not happy to see physicians. Her fear just melted away because of your pleasant approach and your calming personality. **She noticed less pain after her FIRST visit**. She is now coming on a weekly basis to maintain her much improved condition.

PAUL GOLDEBERG, Allamuchy, NJ sales

I can't thank you enough for your treatment of my ailing right shoulder. I had very restricted mobility of my right arm, following a snowboarding accident. Whatever movement I did have was accompanied by chronic pain. Under your expert care, however, I now have full use of my arm and shoulder. I'm lifting weights again, playing weekend softball, and have even been able to start my swimming workouts in preparation for a triathlon this summer. I am a very satisfied and grateful patient. I'm now a true believer in the power of chiropractic care.

KENNETH D. INADOMI, New York, NY, entrepreneur

I had chronic lower back pain, leg pain, and headaches for 4 years. I had seen 5 doctors, took many medications, and was on disability for a year and a half. **After approximately 3 weeks of chiropractic treatments, the headaches and leg pain were gone**. Although the lower back pain still comes once in a while, it has subsided a considerable amount.

STEVEN LEONARDO, Panther Valley, NJ business

I think coming to this office was the best thing for me. They are friendly and caring there. I feel so much better; I had this pain for 7 years. I feel so much better with Dr Fedich's care, thank you!

LINDA ERLING, Allamuchy, NJ, bank teller

My pain would wake me up causing loss of sleep, my neck pain had progressed into my left arm, throughout the treatments and the doctor listening to me, I felt that my condition would improve and it did!

EILEEN MCCABE, Hackettstown, NJ, realtor

I was moving a refrigerator and I pinched a nerve in my back, I couldn't even stand for a few hours, **doctor Fedich saw me the same day, <u>and I got relief!</u>** Within three visits I got total relief and was back to work.

RANDY WANOUS MANSFIELD, NJ, Mansfield school maintenance

There was a significant improvement in my level of pain, **I felt less anxious and more happy!**

ROSE WINZINGER, Independence, NJ

When I was a regular patient, **I was rarely sick**!

JEFF ROSEQUIST, Green Twsp teacher

Dr Jim and Staff, thank you from **everyone here at WNTI 91.9 FM!**

MELANIE THIEL, WNTI radio personality, centenary college, NJ

I had pain in my lower back through my hips and down the top of my thighs. I had lost range of motion bending from the hips and twisting from side to side. I had these problems for over a year. I saw an orthopedic sports doctor, pain management and would take ibuprofen daily. **After my MUA in February 2009, my range of motion came back immediately and the pain in my hips and thighs was gone by the last day! Chiropractic care enables me to continue to dance effectively!**

PAT LANCIANO, Byram, NJ, dance instructor.

I give you Dr Fedich full credit for my current health and well being, I am now able to take care of my newborn baby. **I have no more pain and can take care of my son**!

EMY SMITH, Allamuchy, mother

Dr Fedich is fantastic! He really helped me to be able to live pain free. His treatments are definitely beneficial. I used to have shoulder, neck and back pain, no more!

BRIAN REIFSTECK, Blairstown, Nj, Cadbury Corp

I had a herniated disc in my spine, **I could not work, sleep, or move... after 4 visits my pain was gone and my posture had improved!**

PATTI HAAR, Hackettstown, NJ denial hygienist

I had pain for nine years after having two severe auto accidents, **I had seen 7 doctors** and took too many medications, I did not have a normal life because of the pain and medications. After Dr. Fedich's chiropractic treatments, and Manipulation under anesthesia, I have been feeling better. I can walk like a normal person, do my housework, and play with my grandchildren. I truly feel like a new person. **Thanks god for Dr Fedich**!

DELORIS BROWN, Hackettstown, NJ retired

I had trouble **sleeping, standing, and walking due to my lower back pains.** I am so glad I decided to come here because I feel like I can do all my normal activities that I was unable to do before.

KELLY KUPSTKA, Belvidere, NJ, business

I had lower back pain, middle back pain and stiffness for two years. I had a difficult time bending and reaching for things, after 6 visits I was able to bend and move much easier. My pain is gone and I am doing exercise, I feel great!

STEVEN SQUIRI, Hackettstown, NJ, business owner.

I had lower back pain for 35 years; I had seen many doctors including other chiropractors. I was not able to play golf have been helped a great deal!

ED DRYBURGH HACKETTSTOWN, NJ, owner Dryburgh Piano

On behalf of the International Trace Center Alliance, I would like to extend our thanks and appreciation!

LAURA RIMMER, president international trade center alliance, Mount Olive, NJ

I had back pain for ten years, I couldn't breathe without it hurting, now all the activities I perform are pain-free. **The service was invaluable**; I perform manual labor and wouldn't be able to perform my duties without the treatments!

MIC CALOUCIO, Stanhope, NJ, landscaper

On Behalf of the residents of the House of the Good Sheppard, I would like to thank you!

CHRISTINE GAROFALO, House of Good Sheppard Retirement Community, Hackettstown, NJ

On behalf of Norswescap food bank, we would like to extend our sincerest thanks to you for your participation in our food drive, your generous donation of over 300 lbs of food is greatly appreciated.

BECKY BROOKING, CATHY RUMMELS, directors, Norwescap Food Bank, Phillipsburg, NJ

I had heard several positive things about Dr Fedich before I first met him. During my initial consultation **I found Dr Fedich to be personable, dedicated healer**. He listened patiently as I described what I was experiencing and he assured me that he could help and indeed he has. I would encourage anyone considering chiropractic care to speak with Dr Fedich and begin to receive relief from chronic pain at the hands of a skilled physician.

JAMES SIMMONS, Hackettstown, NJ, guidance counselor

I hurt my back at work on a Friday afternoon and was in a great deal of pain. I was scheduled to run in a triathlon on early Sunday morning. I needed to get help right away. Within twenty minutes of leaving a message on your machine, you called me up and made a special appointment for me. You can came in on your day off and saw me within the next hour. You spent twenty minutes with me, and I was feeling much better. I am please to say that I woke up the next morning pain-free and had an excellent competition. In fact, I achieve a personal record on the course and knocked 43 minutes off last years time! It was a glorious day. Thank you very much for going out of your way to see me and thank you for doing such a good job, **without your**

help I am not sure I would have been able to compete. I will not forget what you did for me!

JEFF DEVINE, Hackettstown, NJ, **triathlete**

I had back pain for several years and tried many chiropractic treatments. However **after my MUA my pain was completely gone for the first time in years!**

RANDY RANDAZZO, Hackettstown, NJ laborer.

Special Offers!

Offer one

If you live in North West New Jersey, and would like a chance to meet Dr Fedich, we are offering a limited time special for anyone who reads my book. We are offering an initial consultation, full examination and digital spinal examination, a full workup, for absolutely nothing! Totally Free, just call the main office number at 908-813-8200, and **mention Docs book**, and we will schedule special time for you meet with Dr. Fedich and see if you have a problem he may be able to help you with. Dr Fedich cant help everyone, but isn't it worth the chance to find out, for no charge! This service usually costs 150 dollars, and will only be **available for free** for book readers for a limited time. By federal law, this offer must exclude Medicare and Medicaid patients. We would still love you to come in and see us though!

Offer two

Do you work for a small to large sized company who may be interested in improving workplace safety, lessen work related injuries, or provide OSHA mandated safety training? Dr. Fedich is an experience health coach and speaker. If your interested in booking Dr. Fedich for a lecture, health talk or as a safety counselor, please call the main office number at 908-813-8200, mention this book, and Dr. Fedich will provide a free phone or in person consultation to discuss your needs

For More Information on Dr Fedich, chiropractic care or his offices, please contact:
Email: Dr. James Fedich drfedich@villagefamilychiro.com
Web   http://www.villagefamilychiro.com
Phone: (908) 813-8200
Main Office Location:
1510 Route 517
Panther Valley Mall
Allamuchy, NJ 07820
Other Locations as well, call the main office for more detail.

Made in the USA
Charleston, SC
01 July 2012